Varicose Veins, Related Diseases and Sclerotherapy:

A Guide for Practitioners

by H.I. Biegeleisen

Eden Press
Montréal · London

VARICOSE VEINS, RELATED DISEASES AND SCLEROTHERAPY: A GUIDE FOR PRACTITIONERS

H.I. Biegeleisen, M.D.

4626 St. Catherine St. West
Montreal, Quebec, Canada H3Z 1S3
and
3 Henrietta Street
London WC2E 8LU England

ISBN: 0-920792-18-9

Credits:
Cover photo: Artery vein, J.F. Gennaro,
L.R. Grillone, Photo Researchers Inc., New York
Cover Design: J.W. Stewart
Text Production: Kathleen Kryklywy

Printed In Canada at Imprimerie Gagné Ltée.
Dépôt légal – première trimestre 1984
Bibliothèque nationale du Québec

TABLE OF CONTENTS

LIST OF ILLUSTRATIONS

PART ONE: VARICOSE VEINS AND RELATED DISEASES

PART TWO: SCLEROTHERAPY

Gratefully dedicated to my wife,
Dorothy,
who made this book possible.

PREFACE

Books are often introduced apologetically by their authors. I offer no such apology. This volume fills a void in our medical knowledge. It describes an important new field and had to be written.

After more than half a century of creative work and intensive research in this area, I find the subjects of varicose veins, its complications, and sclerotherapy largely unrecognized and also grossly misunderstood.

While many physicians employ some of the techniques described herein, few recognize that they are practicing methods related to each other. They are not aware that when assembled, this work becomes an important new branch of medicine requiring special knowledge, training, and skill for its practice. In other words, it is a new specialty although I have been employing it for fifty-five years.

As the pioneer worker in all the phases of sclerotherapy, I feel it is my responsibility to consolidate and record the evolution of this art so it can be studied, taught, and utilized appropriately. This book can act as a guide and reference work for this purpose.

As new methods were added to the original techniques, it became necessary to identify this work by an appropriate name. Thus, *sclerotherapy* was coined by me in 1936 for this purpose when it was used for the first time as the name of the injection clinic at the Stuyvesant Polyclinic in New York City. The idea for the name came from the extension of the sclerosing principle used in varicose veins to other areas of the body.

Sclero, which means to harden, joined to *therapy* describes the process perfectly. It is a fibrosing or hardening of the tissues resembling the end result of surgery.

While working in this pioneer clinic, I reported numerous injection advances, and in 1940 a paper entitled "Sclerotherapy" was published in *Clinical Medicine and Surgery*. These early reports established the name of the specialty as sclerotherapy. Other workers who followed also reported on their progress in this field until the name became accepted world-wide as a designation for sclerosing injection methods.

Curiously enough, this book was first written by me forty years ago at the request of a leading medical publisher,* who wanted a monograph solely on varicose veins. I complied with his request, but never offered it for publication, because it was soon rendered obsolete by the rapid progress in this field. I, therefore, described the individual techniques in a series of reports published in leading medical journals both here and abroad.

Following this, in a veritable information explosion, an enormous bibliography arose because of the many conditions which were yielding to the syringe. The literature on the subject constantly increased.

Today there are societies engaged in its study in most advanced countries. Also, the International Union of Phlebological and Angiological Societies conducts annual conventions for the purpose of discussing the latest developments in this new field of medicine.

The numerous procedures assembled and described herein were created and introduced over a fifty year span. Although my techniques, among others, are now accepted therapy, they were not recognized as either innovations or "breakthroughs" when originally described.

The book is divided into two parts. The first part deals with varicose veins, its complications, and related diseases. The second part describes sclerotherapy and its offshoot, prolotherapy. There is a chapter on future developments of sclerotherapy, some of which have had preliminary testing.

It is hoped that this volume will stimulate the long overdue interest of medical schools and hospitals in these procedures and to include them in their teaching and training programs. Medical school graduates, resident physicians, and many practitioners are handicapped by a lack of knowledge regarding this work because there is still no organized teaching program. As a result, there are not sufficient clinics with the special equipment and trained staffs needed to treat the enormous number of patients who could be helped without surgery. It is estimated that for varicose veins alone in the United States, at least fifteen percent of the population is afflicted, making the number of cases an astounding thirty million.

This is the first manual of its kind which deals with all the sclerosing techniques as a coherent group of procedures now recognized as sclerotherapy. Increasing the widespread practice of this new specialty would reduce the morbidity and mortality of these diseases.

---

* Later became Grune and Stratton

PART ONE ■ VARICOSE VEINS AND RELATED DISEASES

Chapter 1

■ VARICOSE VEINS

Varicose veins is a widespread chronic disease which has been neglected because of its apparently trivial nature and harmless appearance. It cannot be cured permanently in most cases because it is the result of genetically induced weak fascia. This weakness consistently follows hereditary lines and cannot be extirpated by any existing therapy. Yet treatment, which is often neglected because of the simplistic appearance of the disease, should be carried out in most cases as will be demonstrated later. This chapter introduces the concept of varicose veins and its rational treatment which I have developed after more than a half century of intensive study and practice in this field.

Varicose veins are enlarged and stretched blood vessels that are tortuous or irregularly twisted in a characteristic fashion. Their valve flaps no longer meet anatomically to keep the blood flowing normally in one direction, namely, toward the heart. They are present only in humans being practically unknown in animals.*

This disease is the price the human race is paying for standing up on its hind legs, walking on hard pavements, and wearing shoes.

The human body has not kept pace with evolution by adaptation, and its fascial system, which includes venous walls is suffering. The vascular system, and indeed the whole lower extremity, has degenerated and weakened. Thus, ill-adapted in its modern environment, mutations resulting in inherited weaknesses have developed to cause many sagging defects, among which varicose veins are an outstanding example.

The whole subject of fascial weakness will be discussed more fully later in Part 2, Chapter 15. However, at this point, it will suffice to report that these well marked hereditary patterns are very noticeable in afflicted family groups and are a major etiologic factor in varicose veins which is not sufficiently emphasized.

---

*Personal communication – Directors, New York and Bronx Zoos.

It is of paramount importance to recognize the basic fact that we are dealing with a developmental genetic weakness which can now only be alleviated, but not permanently removed by any treatment method. Understanding this, it becomes obvious that the never ending dispute over which therapy produces the best result comes from a lack of this fundamental understanding. Relapses, and even complete regrowth of varicosities cannot be eliminated permanently by any known technique, including compression sclerotherapy, because other veins will inevitably enlarge and become varicosed. In other words, we are dealing with a chronic disease. This is a radically new concept and will be discussed fully in Chapter 11.

Factors which spur the formation of varicose veins in these susceptible individuals are occupation, sex, improper shoes, phlebitis, pregnancy, and obesity.

The conservative therapists utilizing injection methods continue to clash with surgical technicians. Each group claims better results when, in fact, neither has arrived at a perfect solution. Within these groups themselves, failure is often ascribed to improper technique with insufficient reference to the actual primordial cause of inherited fascial deficiency.

The treatment concept which I advocate utilizes all the reported successful sclerosing techniques, followed by periodic annual check-ups. This will control the disease and even produce apparent cures in mild cases where the fascial structure is only slightly affected by hereditary predisposition. In my opinion, it becomes the treatment of choice.

Anatomy

A knowledge of the anatomy of the venous system of the lower extremities is needed in order to perform this work. Aside from the relations and distribution of the lesser and greater saphenous systems of veins, the important things to be aware of are the communicating veins, the valves, the structure of the vein walls, and the satellite veins. These will now be summarized.

Communicating Veins

These perforator veins penetrate the muscles and their fascia to connect superficial with deep veins in the leg and thigh. Usually there are two branches in the middle and lower thigh (sometimes none). In the lower leg they are very frequent and scattered. They have been intensively studied and their patterns described by Sherman (1).

Valves

They are present in the superficial, deep and communicating veins. The valve cusps face inward and upward preventing the reflux of blood and, thereby, maintaining the blood column above them. They are commonly near the opening of a tributary and distal to it.

Valves are usually bicuspid, while many are unicuspid and occasionally tricuspid. Most bicuspids are in the saphenous veins and also in the deep veins of the lower leg.

Satellite Veins and Venae Comitantes

Along the main trunks of the small or large saphenous veins in both thighs and legs are often found small normal veins parallel to them. These tiny veins may enlarge after successfully closing the main veins. Some patients are then led to believe that the original vein *came back* when, in reality, the varicose development is due to this anatomic finding. Satellite veins and venae comitantes may also accompany smaller varicose veins and may similarly enlarge after apparently perfect therapy.

Etiology

Other theories regarding the etiology of varicose veins have been proposed which deserve mention.

There is a loss of valves from birth to adult life due to back pressures. Investigators have found there are many more valves present at birth then persist in adult life, which may be a factor in development of varicosities. Injury to valves as a result of phlebitis is an accepted precursor of varicose development. Pregnancy, with its increased venous pressure in the lower limbs, and hormonal influences are also accepted causes of varicose veins, which often correct themselves spontaneously in the months following childbirth. Occupational factors in individuals who stand excessively predisposes to varicosities, because these individuals lack the beneficial pumping effect of muscular contractions. Sex factors are equal up to the age of twenty, after which the proportion of women to men with varicose veins is about four to one.

All the above etiologic reasons may be regarded as exciting causes acting upon a hereditary faulty genetic constitution. Otherwise it would be difficult to explain why some individuals never develop varicosities under any circumstances. This tremendous hereditary influence has been amply noted and documented by me in over fifty-five years of highly active peripheral vascular practice.

Compensatory veins are varicosities, which sometimes result from a deep venous thrombosis, which has caused transient blockage of the deep venous system. My x-ray studies, which will be discussed later, have demonstrated the absence of permanent deep blocking because of the natural development of significant collateral blood vessels that I have demonstrated radiographically (2). Thus, any *deep block* may be regarded as relative, rather than absolute. During this compensatory phase, however, varicose veins may develop in the superficial venous system.

Another unusual condition is arteriovenous shunt or fistula. Here a direct union occurs between the arteries and veins, often soon after birth. It has been claimed without sufficient confirmation that most varicosities arise in this fashion. It will be more fully discussed.

Obesity is sometimes mentioned as a cause of varicose veins and patients themselves often suggest it. This does not seem to be a real factor, as some of the most advanced cases of varicosities I have observed occurred in very thin individuals.

Organizing Thrombosis

McPheeters (3) in his monograph published in 1938, was the first author to demonstrate by a series of fluoroscopic studies, following the injection of radio-opaque Lipiodol solution, that the circulation in varicose veins was either stagnant or actually reversed. Noting that, normally, all venous flow is upward, he showed that in the varicose limb, the injected Lipiodol globules were seen to flow downward or remain stationary. This was an important new concept.

The biggest change in our thinking in this era lies in the fact that we have come to recognize the menace of producing large, bulky thromboses by the sclerosing method. While the incidence of pulmonary embolism with modern injection treatment of varicose veins has become insignificant, it is now recognized that *empty vein* techniques which produce much smaller or no thrombi, reduce still further the hazard of treating large varicosities by modern sclerotherapy. Any detached clot is usually forced distally toward the branching and smaller veins where it is arrested.

The sclerosing process has been demonstrated to produce an organizing thrombosis which is attached to the vein wall where it undergoes a series of pathologic changes ending up in a fibrous occlusion.

Modern sclerotherapy, with its latest refinement of empty-vein techniques and compression bandaging, improves this picture by aiming as often as possible in producing wall to wall intimal primal fibrosis. When achieved, this primary fibrotic closure of the vein is the utopia of injection aims, and makes the treatment of varicose veins more efficient than ever before. However, each case has to be handled individually. A judicious operator will know from experience that it is not possible to do an entire complicated case solely by one type of injection, but rather each vein requires individual appraisal and handling. This will be described in the chapter on injection treatment. I find that older, stand-up techniques are by no means to be discarded completely.

Differential Diagnosis

The differential diagnosis of varicose veins is simple, because it is usually made by observation alone. A varicose vein is a characteristic venous enlargement that cannot be confused with anything else. However, patients frequently ask whether the smallest venous enlargements, which are called venules, are also part of the varicose vein picture. These vessels are unacceptable to many patients, because they stand out as bluish to purplish lines on normal skin. Some of these venules are normal vessels, other are varicose. Sensitive individuals often request their removal for cosmetic reasons.

Venules

Venules are borderline enlargements. They are not twisted, but are sometimes the first stage of small varicose vein formation. They may cause painful symptoms, because the tiny blood vessels are in the first stage of stretching which compresses nerve endings in the skin. When they become larger, the pain often disappears, a phenomenon that has to be explained to the patient. They are also influenced by the amount of fluid in the body, so that prior to menstruation, when the body fluid is at its maximum volume, the little blood vessels are more conspicuous. At other times, they are less evident or, indeed, absent. For successful treatment, dilated venules must be dealt with at the appropriate time, when they are readily observable. This can only be done in the stand-up position.

Blotches

In some individuals, bluish to purplish discoloration, best described by the term *blotching*, is found often accompanying capillary enlargements. They are readily blanched by pressure which usually establishes the diagnosis.

Blotches vary in size from tiny spots up to areas several inches in diameter. They may occur without any varicosities at all, and may then be considered a type of angioma. When they are found accompanying capillary enlargements or small varicose veins, there is a good chance that they may disappear after the completion of treatment for the varicosities or surrounding capillaries. The treatment of blotches is described in "Cosmetic Aspects" (Chapter 14).

Arteriovenous Shunts

As noted, the diagnosis of varicose veins is usually simple. However, in the presence of arteriovenous shunting, as previously described, there may be confusion. This abnormal development is due to a direct union between the arteries and veins. It may occur in either the arm or leg and is often diagnosed as a case of congenital varicose veins, because it was present at birth or was noticed soon afterwards.

An accurate diagnosis can be made by comparing the oxygen content of the varicose blood with that in the normal veins of the same individual. Sometimes, the venous blood in this condition is a bright red color like that in arterial blood. This condition responds poorly to injection treatment which will call attention to the special nature of the problem. Treatment in these cases must be evaluated individually, as sometimes surgery is a necessity. Conversely, there may be instances where injection treatment will gradually control the condition, if surgery fails.

The symptoms of varicose veins are not uniform and cannot be depended upon for diagnosis in all cases. Thus, many fortunate individuals with advanced varicose conditions may go for a lifetime without serious symptomatology. Varicose veins usually is not a painful disease; however, most patients will state that their legs feel heavy, the varicose areas are hot, and that they suffer from frequent cramps in bed at night. Less commonly, cramps occur during the daytime, if their occupation requires long standing. They will be uncomfortable due to the heaviness or swelling of the afflicted limb. In the presence of complications like ulcer or phlebitis, the picture changes and pain becomes a prominent symptom.

The operator will be called upon to differentiate other conditions which have symptoms resembling varicose veins. One of these is Raynaud's disease.

Raynaud's Disease

This disease, which presents changes in color, is often limited to the toes and fingers. It may occur in the absence or presence of varicose veins, and is directly influenced by the temperature of the environment. The symptoms are precipitated by cold temperatures; there are no cramps.

The usual syndrome that establishes the diagnosis of Raynaud's consists of periods of blanching, alternating with intervals of reddish or purple discoloration. There may be phases of color changes depending on the skin temperature. Thus, an individual may note on a cold day that his hands or feet become blanched in the exposed areas. With warmth the blanching may be replaced by normal coloration. The best way to explain Raynaud's disease to patients is to describe it as an imbalance of the vasomotor mechanism in the terminal blood vessels of the hands or feet. Thus, while a balanced terminal vascular system imparts a normal flesh tone to the skin, the lack of balance in Raynaud's disease permits one set of fibers, the vasoconstrictors, which constrict the blood vessels, to overpower the other muscle fibers, called the vasodilators, or vice versa, causing the various color changes. With vasoconstrictors in control, the skin color is white; while with vasodilators the color is cyanotic or purplish. The condition occurs mostly in younger women with only 5% of cases present in men.

Primary Erythromelalgia

Another condition to be differentiated because of disturbed skin color is primary erythromelalgia. This disease occurs in both sexes equally, and is seen rarely in peripheral vascular practice. It is characterized by paroxysmal bilateral vasodilation, causing what the name implies, red legs. It usually affects the feet, rather than the hands, causing burning pain and increased skin temperature with marked redness of the skin. This condition is not easily confused with varicose veins.

Buerger's Disease

Buerger's disease (endarteritis obliterans) seems to be diminishing in frequency as the years go by. This may be a reflection of the lessened use of tobacco as a result of public education. It is characterized by its prevalence in Hebrew males (99%). This condition in advanced cases ultimately restricts the peripheral arterial flow to the extremities, with the development of gangrene. About one-third of the cases exhibit migrating phlebitis, which is a diagnostic aid. Clinically, the arterial impairment can be demonstrated by the oscillometer and Doppler machines. Thus, there is no problem in making the differential diagnosis.

Low-Back Syndrome

The physician working on varicose veins must also be alert to the frequent occurrence of pain in the lower limbs. This is less often due to varicose veins and more often due to referred pain as part of the low-back syndrome. The diagnosis is frequently missed because the original back injury may have taken place as much as twenty years ago. In fact, the patient may have completely forgotten the initial attack.

It is not generally known that relapses of low-back attacks can occur without causing any backache. Instead, the patients experience referred leg pains, which utterly confuse them and, often, their physicians. Back injuries, frequently do not heal well and are subject to repeated relapses. They may then continue to exhibit painful radiation down the lower extremities in a confusing pattern.

In these instances experienced physicians will be guarded in their prognosis of pain relief from vein treatment. This will be discussed in more detail in the chapter on low-back syndrome (Chapter 21).

Arthritides

A large group of diseases which may confuse the operator, again because of the leg symptoms, are the arthritides.

Pain in the leg, occurring in individuals who have both varicose veins and arthritis of the knee, for example, must be appraised carefully before treatment. The doctor must explain to the patient that pain due to arthritis may only occasionally be relieved by correcting the venous stagnation.

The arthritic process, if persistent, may continue to run its course unabated, in spite of venotherapy.

To conclude, the disease of uncomplicated varicose veins is not basically a painful condition and its diagnosis is readily established.

Chapter 2

▪ PREPARATION FOR INJECTION TREATMENT OF VARICOSE VEINS

Equipment

The injection treatment of varicose veins is a precise art. The principles involved and the techniques described herein will guide the operator in his therapy.

Before proceeding with techniques, it is necessary to discuss the equipment used, under their separate headings.

Syringes

Syringes are best in glass with concentric tips. Sizes may vary from ¼ c.c. (tuberculin) to 20 c.c. Most injections are made with a 2 c.c. syringe. Luerlocks are not recommended as they interfere with freedom of motion. Standard-make syringes are advisable.

For the kind of accuracy and handling required in these delicate techniques, nothing equals the glass syringe at this time. However, with the advent of plastic disposable syringes, a whole new armamentarium has been added with special advantages. Namely, they are packaged conveniently sterile, and may be obtained with the needle attached, if desired, so that the nuisance of autoclaving constantly is eliminated.

For various vein techniques, the plastic sterile syringe is a mixed blessing. Its most serious defect is the lack of smooth, precise response with the one-handed operation necessary for the average injection. The operator should have the control needed to draw the plunger back with one or two fingers and aspirate one or more minims accurately, at will, leaving the other hand free for palpation. This cannot be done with the usual plastic syringe as yet, with the exception of the ½ to 1 c.c. sizes.

In these small sizes, the syringes operate with admirable smoothness and can be well controlled with one hand. As the plastic sizes increase to 2 or 3 c.c.

and beyond, sticking of the barrel or inadequate response to aspiration, hinders their effectiveness. Two-handed operation is often necessary.

When it comes to 5, 10, or 20 c.c. syringe sizes, one-handed techniques are not practical with any syringe. Here plastic syringes for two-handed techniques are quite useful, especially when employing catheter needles (see Chapter 3). With these, palpation during injection is not so essential, as the needle, once it is properly inserted and taped into place, is usually safely contained within the vein wall.

The small tuberculin plastic syringe mentioned above (½ to 1 c.c.), because of its smooth action on aspiration and injection, is uniquely suitable for venule and capillary injections (see Chapter 13).

Needles

The story of needles is long and never-ending because there are always new types being introduced. The latest additions are the disposable needles of various sizes. They now comprise a large group of great diversity. However, one fact never changes and that is that the needle point can never be too sharp or too pointed for vein work.

In earlier years, workers in this field used to sharpen their own needle points by hand. This was accomplished by electrified grinding wheels to create the desired bevel, which was then honed on oil stones. Manufacturer's needles were often not sharp enough for the exacting requirements of varicose vein therapy.

Their aim and mine as well was to produce a curved or flat bevel with knife-like edges and a sharp tip. It was found that the longer the bevel, the sharper one could make the point. Nurses and doctors spent hours cleaning, sharpening, and styleting the needles they used over and over again. All burrs were carefully removed on very fine oil stones. It was a never-ending struggle to personally fashion needle points, as perfectly as possible for increased accuracy in injection technique.

A new era in needle making developed when the disposable needle with a bayonet point was developed which, in addition to a very sharp tip, had side bevels with four cutting edges. These needles entered the skin and veins with little effort beyond a slight stabbing motion, and met with wide acceptance for routine medical use and also for varicose vein work.

It was a momentous advance, because it relieved the doctor and his staff of much tedious work. These needles were not only disposable and inexpensive, but did not require sterilization or cleaning. However, machine made disposable needles were not always perfect, and some of them came to the doctor either clogged or burred.

Most of the imperfect ones could be weeded out when the solutions were drawn up prior to use. Nevertheless, even with occasional imperfections it was advantageous in varicose vein practice to have sharp, sterilized needles always available.

When used with glass syringes, the doctor has available a tool of very practical efficiency. Generally, long bevels are preferable in this field of injection work, because this makes for a longer and sharper point. But there is the disadvantage of more frequent burring, because as the point gets longer, the tip becomes thinner and more readily bent. Needless to say, a burred tip will hardly ever enter a vein properly, if it gets in at all. It is also more painful for the patient.

When it comes to fine, tiny vessel injections, such as we find in telangiectasia (capillary dilatations), a special, very minute needle has to be employed. I have developed the finest and most delicate needle (gauge 33) in the peripheral vascular field and the micro-techniques involved in its use (4) are learned only by assiduous and repeated practice (Chapter 12).*

Catheter Needles

The use of catheter needles for sclerotherapy has been a boon to this art. Originally intended for hospital use during intravenous therapy, they are manufactured disposable and sterilized for immediate use. These needles are now regularly employed for the treatment of special varicose vein techniques. They are of two types: The Butterfly Infusion Needle and catheter, and the teflon styleted catheter needles.

The Butterfly Infusion Needle comes in various sizes, with a most useful 19 gauge suitable for the saphenous vein. The soft plastic catheter attached to it terminates in a hub that can receive a syringe containing sclerosing fluid (Fig. 1).

The intravenous catheter placement units with teflon catheters and stylets can be obtained in 20 and 22 guage sizes and are made of two parts. One is the catheter containing the needle inside, and the other is just the stylet attached to a hub (Fig. 2). Their use in described later under empty vein techniques (Chapters 4 and 5).

* Commercially, gauges 30, 31, 32 and 33 are available but are inferior to custom made needles. The 30 guage size is disposable.

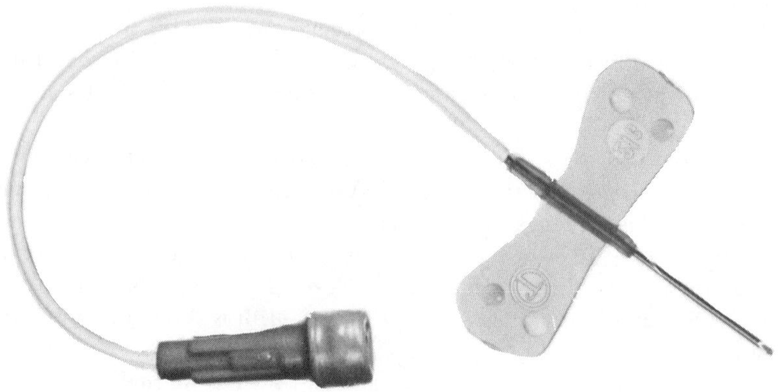

Figure 1. Butterfly infusion needle

Diagnostic Aids

It is only occasionally that it becomes necessary to perform venography as an aid in evaluating the superficial varicose and deep venous circulation (see Chapter 12). The x-ray technique which I introduced in 1939 (5) was intended for the differential diagnosis of the various forms of unilateral enlargement of the lower extremity. My studies indicated that there is rarely any contra-indication to injection treatment of varicose veins even in the presence of inequality in size between the lower limbs.

Comparatively recent developments in the Doppler ultrasonic method of studying circulatory flow in the deep vascular system has added a new instrument for the study of blood flow circulation. By the aid of this machine, the presence or absence of venous flow can be evaluated by direct auscultation. Characteristic sounds are heard by placing a pressure sensor on the skin lying over a blood vessel which enables the operator to estimate the velocity of blood flow beneath the applicator, to a depth of 5 cms. Conversion of the ultrasonic signals into an electric circuit with subsequent amplification as an audio signal enables the operator to actually hear the blood flow.

With recent refinement in technique, it is now possible to determine whether a deep vein is open or closed and an estimate can be made of the degree of such closure. The audio signals can also aid in differentiating between the pumping sounds of arterial flow and the rushing wind noises heard in the deep venous system. Where a vein and an artery lie in close relationship with each other, identifying sounds will disclose both blood vessels. The Doppler

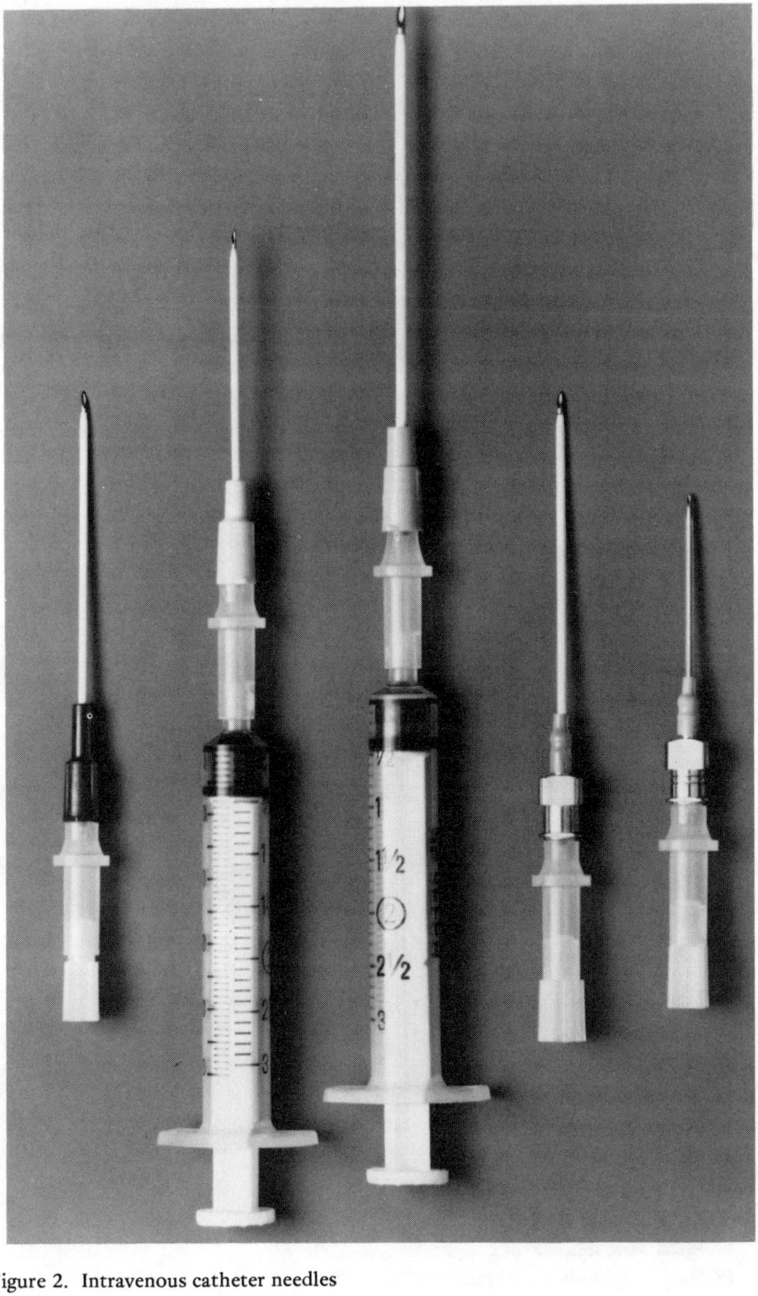

Figure 2. Intravenous catheter needles

ultrasonic method of studying blood vessel flow is an added confirmatory sign to what the experienced operator can ascertain by the usual means of physical diagnosis.

Illumination

Working light should be of the daylight type. It must be strong, even and diffuse. This is not always available indoors and so a bank of artificial lights must be provided giving this kind of illumination whenever needed. For consistent results the operator should always use the same lighting rather than switch from artificial light to natural light. The latter is confusing for accuracy. Sunlight shining directly on the patient is rarely satisfactory.

Special operating lights with intense shadow-free illumination will be needed for the micro-injection technique of capillary injections. Sometimes illuminated magnifiers on portable floor stands are useful for the delicate techniques involved for dilated venules.

Position of the Patient

For the average upright technique described later, the author's own vein table designed fifty years ago is still the most useful (Fig. 3). This consists of

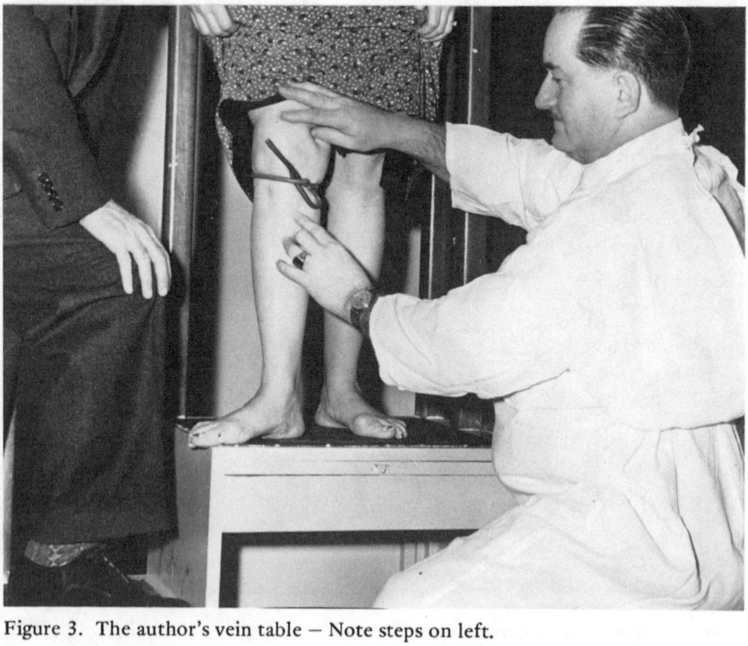

Figure 3. The author's vein table – Note steps on left.

a sturdy table 27 to 29 inches high, with two steps leading to the top. There should be a handrail for the steps and an upright pole for the patient to hold onto during the treatment. The operator sits in front of this table and should be able to reach any part of the lower extremity comfortably while seated.

The patient may also sit on this table for treatment, with the legs hanging down, horizontal or raised up. The latter position is favored for empty-vein techniques. Thus, there are three positions which may be assumed by the patient while sitting on this treatment table.

For the more precise treatment of capillary dilatations, a motorized operating table is needed to allow for changes in height and angle of the patients' limbs. This table is also needed for the various empty-vein techniques involving the great saphenous vein and its branches.

Slowing the Venous Blood Flow

The venous blood flow in varicose veins is often slow, stagnant, or reversed, making it an ideal situation for sclerotherapy, which depends upon chemical irritation of the intima. However, some large veins, especially when associated with muscular perforators or *blow-outs* have a more rapid blood stream. Here it becomes essential to further slow the flow, so that the sclerosing fluid can better act upon the intimal lining.

This was recognized early in the author's experience and various devices were in vogue at that time. These included a malleable lead wire occluder, the Cohen vascular clamp and various tourniquets. The older rubber tube tourniquets have been largely displaced in recent years by the newer *velcro* self-adhering types. Also, the operator's finger techniques, which were always useful in localizing the injection reaction by judicious finger pressure, are still in use.

Bandages and Compression

Before commencing treatment, physicians employing this technique must prepare themselves with elastic bandages, foam rubber sponges, and be conversant with the use of special support stockings. These are finding increasing use for compression sclerotherapy, which emphasizes continuous support bandaging and concentrated injections (Chapter 5). The theory is that recanalization of thrombosed veins may occur more readily, unless the entire limb is swathed in bandages with soft cotton pressure balls or other elastic sponges which are fixed over the injected sites. This will be discussed in its proper place below.

For the usual stand-up technique which is still an important part of sclerotherapy for varicose veins, the operator must provide himself with pre-cut strips of adhesive tape one inch wide and twelve inches long. These strips are used to hold sterilized ball-shaped gauze sponges in place over the vein that has been treated. The adhesive should be flesh-colored to make it less conspicuous. As many varieties as possible should be available, in order to give the operator sufficient latitude in the event the patient is allergic or sensitive to one or more of the adhesive tapes.

Sometimes, in the overly sensitive individual, it becomes necessary to use paper or industrial tapes. The operator's ingenuity may be sorely tested by some patients who seemingly cannot tolerate any of the usual tapes available. It may then be necessary to bandage the patient with gauze or other material or to use elastic adhesive (Elastoplast)* if all else fails. If the operator is ingenious enough, he will always find some way of maintaining the pressure on a treated varicose vein for a sufficiently long time, (up to 6 weeks according to some observers).

Syringe Grips

There is a basic difference between routine intravenous injection and the special technique necessary for varicose veins. Due to the tortuosity of the varicosed blood vessel, the needle point must be more accurately placed within the vein lumen. Every doctor performs intravenous injections routinely, which he usually learns easily in his hospital training. The technique for varicose veins, however, is on a different order, because not only are the veins tortuous, but they are found in a wide range of sizes, shapes, locations, and pathologic states. Thus veins may be very small and superficial, as in the ankle area, a little larger and deeper in the lower skin layers, or quite large and deeply placed through the fascia covering the muscles, as in the case of perforator veins.

Furthermore, the veins that are treated may be thin walled, of average thickness, or more thickened from inflammatory reactions. They may also be toughened by thickening of the walls as the result of fibrosis or actual calcification. Their sensitivity is also variable depending upon the vein and the patient. It is evident that the operator must develop a flexible technique to suit such a wide range of conditions.

He must learn special ways of grasping and holding the syringe. These will be described as *grips.* Also, in making the actual injection, after entering the vein, he must usually change his grip in order to drive the plunger into the barrel of the syringe. This is shown as *change of grip*.

* BDF Beiersdorf Inc. South Norwalk, Connecticut, 06854.

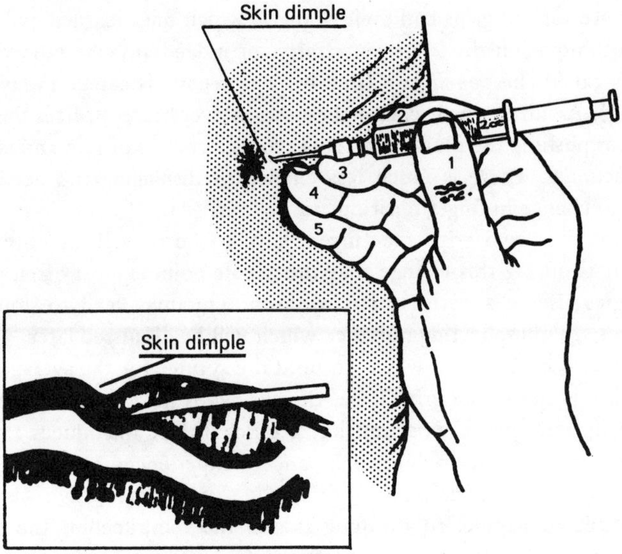

Figure 4. Pencil grip; skin dimple.

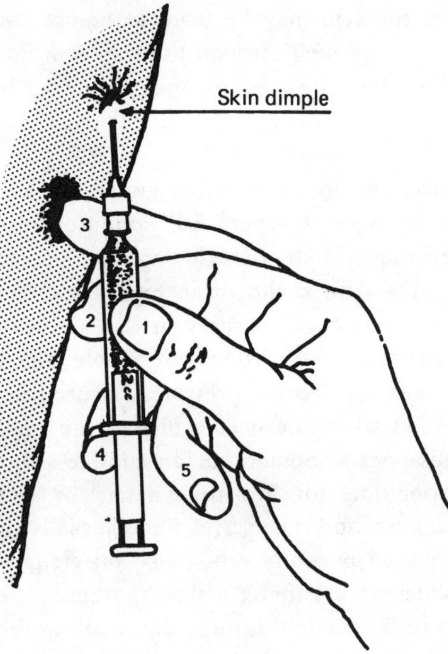

Figure 5. Violin bow grip. Note dimple as injection guide.

There are various grips and their changes, which once learned, will suit any varicose technique on the lower extremity, or indeed anywhere on the body. The first is called the *pencil grip* (Fig. 4). The second is named the *violin-bow grip* (Fig. 5). A third, which cannot be used in every case, utilizes the palm of the hand for pushing the plunger in. This avoids a change of grip and is the best one for accuracy. There is much less chance of displacing the needle point, if there is no change in finger position.

With the first two grips the fingers have to be moved, as noted on the diagrams. It is during this change that the needle point is most often displaced and may give rise to a perivascular injection. This may lead to sloughing or tissue necrosis, a complicating nuisance which will be discussed later.

The most useful way in which to hold the syringe for the average varicose vein injection is the *pencil grip.* Here, the syringe is held as though it were an actual pencil, and with a wrist motion a quick thrust introduces the needle through the skin. Rapidity reduces pain, and an experienced operator can make the sensation of the needle point enterng the skin imperceptible. Usually the needle is directed parallel to the long axis of the vein, keeping the bevel up. This is important, because the bevel deflects the needle point downward below the skin surface into the vein.

The entry into the vein may be made in one or two motions. First, the initial thrust may be continued through the vein wall into the lumen without stopping. This is ideal. Or, the operator may stop after he has penetrated the skin and then sharply thrusts the needle into the vein cavity as a second more careful motion.

In general, injections are made either visually or by palpation. When the light is good and the vein is superficial, conditions are ideal for the more accurate visual technique. Here the guiding sign of correct entry into the vein is dimpling of the skin, as shown on Figs. 4 and 5. It will be noted that as the needle point presses against the vein wall about to be entered, it pulls the skin down in a characteristic little pit or dimple. This is an infallible sign of a perfectly placed injection. As the pressure is continued, there will be a sudden release of tension when the needle pierces the wall of the blood vessel and the dimple disappears. Sometimes an audible snapping sound is heard.

When the lighting does not show these details, or the vein lies more deeply placed, the palpation method is better. A finger, usually the index finger of the opposite hand, is placed over the vein to be injected. Here, as the needle is advanced by a sudden thrust (never a slow movement), entry is indicated by a sudden release of resistance felt through the needle as the vein wall is pierced. The palpating finger is kept in place while the injection is completed. In the event of perivascular injection, a distinct infiltration or whealing will be felt

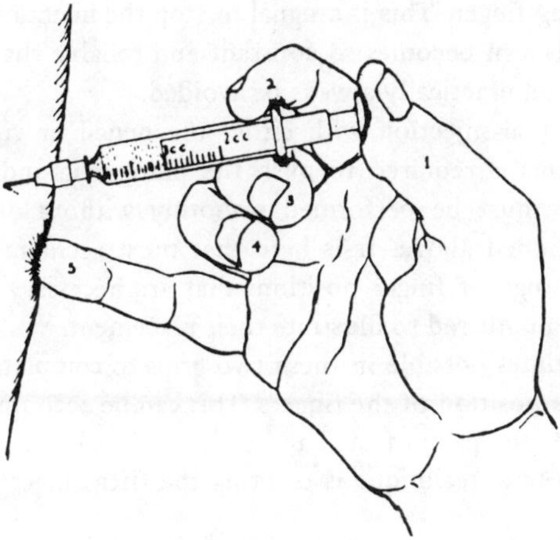

Figure 6. Change of grip for injection. Note fingers are numbered.

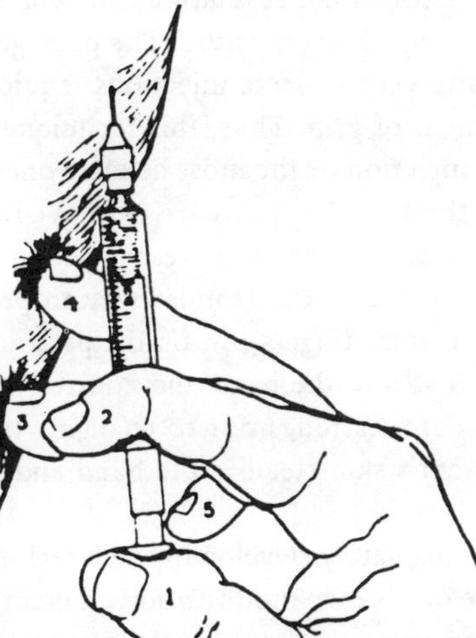

Figure 7. Change of grip for injection. This technique suitable for vertical veins like Great Saphenous.

by the palpating finger. This is a signal to stop the injection immediately. With experience, this sign becomes so constant and reliable that accidental perivascular effusion can practically always be avoided.

For the actual injection with either the pencil or violin-bow technique, a change of grips is required to push the plunger in and inject the solution. This maneuver must be performed smoothly without dislodging the needle point, as mentioned above. It is here that most accidents occur. Figs. 6 and 7 show the change of finger positions that are necessary in order to do this. The fingers are numbered to illustrate their placement.

It is sometimes possible in these two grips to complete the injection without moving the position of the fingers. This can be accomplished with the pencil grip, by using the palm of the hand to force the plunger home. Another way with the violin-bow technique is to bring the fifth finger around to press the plunger in.

The palm grip may sometimes be employed for routine vein injections with a 2 c.c. syringe. It is more difficult technically to perform than the other two grips and is therefore less used. It is also useful where thick, viscous fluids need to be injected, requiring strong pressure. The palm grip, curiously enough, is frequently used for the very delicate injections required in capillary work, in order to avoid a change of grip. Thus, this technique is equally suited for either the most forceful injection or the most delicate one.

For the most part, the first two grips are employed. Reference to Figs. 6 and 7 shows the positions of the fingers are rearranged in each case, so that the thumb can be brought around in the familiar way to press the plunger in. It will be noted that one or more fingers rest on the patient's limb during the injection phase, in order to steady the hand and control the technique. Indeed, even when the injections are started, prior to changing the grip, resting one or more fingers on the patient's skin steadies the hand and adds accuracy to the procedure.

Every operator will ultimately develop his own technique either patterned on those described above or his own modifications thereof.

Some physicians may prefer to simply enter the vein at its most prominent bulge. When I started this work, I cautioned against this type of simplistic approach. I felt that entering the skin first and the vein subsequently was a more scientific procedure, as it protected the vein wall better and prevented a leakage backward of the injected solution. In recent years, I have not been so adamant in my teaching and feel that most beginners get almost as good results by the direct simple technique. Nevertheless, entering the skin first is still the better technique.

Anyone doing this type of venotherapy must train both hands. There are circumstances where the right hand cannot be placed in position for a comforable or accurate injection. Here the opposite hand, if it is properly trained, can often make the injection without any difficulty. Most of the time, however, one trained hand will handle almost all varicose vein injections.

Medical Assistant

It is possible for the family physician to do a simple varicose vein case by himself. However, anyone attempting the modern techniques described herein, for a complicated case or series of cases, will require an assistant for competent treatment. From my extensive clinical experience in this specialized field, I would not attempt this work by myself. There are many occasions when an assistant, and sometimes two, becomes essential for careful work. I prefer working with a nurse stretching and stabilizing the skin to ensure accuracy. Other operators do routine injections without assistants. The individual doctor has to make his own choice.

A tight skin is helpful in these techniques, because one is dealing with veins that are enlarged and moveable with a tendency to evade the point of the needle by sliding in the relaxed skin. With a nurse holding the skin taut, the vein is immobilized and can more readily be penetrated. Indeed, in some areas like the anterior knee, the dorsum of the foot or the ankles, the veins roll aside so readily that two hands, or two assistants, sometimes become necessary. Another difficult area to treat, without proper help, is the scrotal skin area.

The operator is now ready to consider the various solutions used in this treatment.

Chapter 3

▪ SOLUTIONS

History

According to medical historian, Victor Robinson, M.D. (6) sclerosing solutions were first used in 1835 by Velpeau, a French surgeon, who injected a solution of iodine into the hydrocele of a patient, who also had an accompanying hernia. As a result of his injection, both hydrocele and hernia were cured.

The injection treatment of varicose veins, however, was first performed in 1851 by Charles-Gabriel Pravaz of Lyons, with a solution of ferric chloride. It was the same year in which this early worker gave the hypodermic syringe to mankind. There was considerable opposition to this treatment before it became a recognized scientific procedure.

The injection treatment of varicose veins was developed and practiced by early workers in Germany and France who first used concentrated glucose, hypertonic sodium chloride, sodium salicylate, quinine and urethane and bichloride of mercury solutions. These will be described later.

Modern therapy began with the introduction of sodium morrhuate in 1930 when Higgins and Kittel published their epochal article in the *Lancet* (7). This early solution derived from cod-liver oil contains an unknown number of fatty acid salts. It is the parent of a number of sclerosing solutions that followed and is still in use today. The advent of this solution presented the medical profession with an efficient and safe solution for the first time, placing the injection treatment of varicose veins on a widely acceptable basis.

My interest began at this time with a clinical study of sodium morrhuate. Experience soon indicated that this solution was really a liquid soap, containing a mixture of the fatty acids found in cod-liver oil.

At first I duplicated the effects of sodium morrhuate with liquid soap by injecting the ear veins of rabbits and secured thrombosis. Continued testing with 5% sterile sodium oleate, the chief constituent of both cod-liver oil and liquid soap, were similarly successful.

My report of 1933 (8) recommended the isolation and purification of the principal fatty acids found in cod-liver oil, in order to develop standardized pure products for sclerosing therapy.

Leading pharmaceutical companies in America followed these suggestions and developed a series of purified sclerosing agents which were sent to me for testing. I reported on six of these in the medical literature (9, 10). This marked the beginning of the second phase of modern sclerotherapy.

Some of these solutions were merely sodium or potassium salts of vegetable oils which gave rise to sclerosing solutions like *Sylnasol,* made from the oil of psyllium seeds; *Soricin,* derived from castor oil; *ipotole,* made from olive oil; and others.

There were also cumbersome compounds made by combining quinine with these saponified solutions. These were not readily accepted and were soon discontinued. The important sclerosing agents were the purified fatty acid salts like monolate, which were preferred and used widely for about 20 years when their popularity declined due to the introduction of newer, totally synthetic, preparations. The first of these, sodium tetradecyl sulfate, was created by *Riner** originally. The initial test material proved to be too irritating, therefore I recommended a 1% and 3% purified synthetic compound which was finally produced under the name of *Sotradecol* (Table 1). This is the most widely used and efficient sclerosing agent now available.** It has revolutionized sclerotherapy.

It must be pointed out that prior to this, semi-synthetic compounds such as monolate and etalate occasionally caused allergic reactions. While this was puzzling at first, it was explained later by the fact that part of the formula, the oleate fraction, was derived from olive oil which is a natural source and, therefore, contains traces of protein. All of the oleate combinations are subject to a similar contamination. The shift to complete synthesis was an obvious answer to this problem because it helped to avoid allergy.

I pointed out early in my investigations that there is no special chemical magic involved in the development of a sclerosing solution. Almost any safe chemical, and sometimes small amounts of toxic material, can be made to irritate, stimulate, or sclerose human tissue. Thus, a high concentration of normal components of the blood plasma, like sugar or salt, can affect the endothelium of vein walls to produce fibrosis.

Although these substances are constantly present in the blood stream in normal amounts, we are able to make sclerosing solutions out of these bland

---

*Wallace and Tiernan, U.S.A.

**Manufactured and sold in Europe as Trombovar in various strengths.

substances in preparations like invertose 60%, dextrose 50%, or hypertonic saline 18% to 30%.

Obviously, we cannot utilize other fractions of human plasma which are purely excretory products like uric acid and urea.

It will be useful to divide sclerosing solutions into three categories:

1) Solutions made from chemical components found normally in the body like glucose and sodium chloride.

2) Sclerosing solutions made by extracting constituents of plants or animals like the oil of psyllium seeds and cod-liver oil. Refining and purifying these extracts gave rise to a whole series of fatty acid preparations that behaved like liquid soaps to lower surface tension.

3) Solutions that are synthesized partially or completely and are new compounds.

In order to have a clear concept of sclerosing materials, it is not only necessary to understand where they come from, but also how they work.

Modes of Action

1) **Dehydration.** This is typified by the concentrated salts and sugar solutions, which by osmotic action, extract water from the cells in the area of injection, causing injury by dehydration. This starts a series of reactions which causes the special fibrosing clot, to be described later.

2) **Surface Tension Action.** The injected solution produces a *soap effect* which alters the surface tension surrounding the cells under treatment.

3) **Cauterizing Action.** Corrosive solutions used for injection will destroy the cells they contact. This destruction is followed by characteristic fibrosing clots or scar.

4) **Heavy Metal Effect.** This injures the cells in the area to cause tissue injury and clotting.

Postulates for an Ideal Solution

While we have improved sclerosing solutions to such a degree that numerous new techniques have evolved, I feel that in the future a search should be made for an ideal solution through a different pathway. This should be in the biologic or stimulating area instead of our present emphasis on chemical injury and destruction of tissues.

To assist us in this search we must keep in mind the nature of the ideal solution. It should have the following characteristics:

1) Relative freedom from slough formation;

2) Painless on injection;

3) High efficiency as an endothelial and general tissue stimulant,

promoting repair or fibrosis as desired;

4) Non-toxicity in proper dosage;

5) Few, if any, side effects;

6) Purity and standardization of ingredients.

Such an ideal sclerosing agent has not yet been found although we are constantly working toward this goal. It has been, thus far, impossible to develop a chemical irritant that has all these qualities. The problem has been that the tissues involved often have an impoverished blood supply. Minor degrees of chemical irritation can break down the fragile tissues treated because of the borderline circulation. The goal to be achieved is still ideally in the biologic area of development.

Pathology.

The pathological changes following present injection treatment have been extensively studied by McPheeters, Lufkin (11), and others. Most observers reported a special kind of chemical thrombosis following intimal injury. This was followed by an organizing process that converted the vein into a fibrous cord. After disintegration and phagocytosis, absorption took place with shrinking and thinning. Ultimately the cord became converted into a barely palpable string or virtually disappeared. The final result was the clinical removal of the treated varicosity, just as effectively as with surgery.

We know today that the importance of securing primary adhesion between opposing endothelial surfaces was not sufficiently recognized by early workers. With modern empty-vein techniques, which will be described later, the bulky, painful reactions, especially in the larger veins, can today be avoided so that the end results now rival, or in many cases surpass, surgical results. Furthermore, there is no ugly scar left for a condition that usually brings patients to the doctor's office for cosmetic relief. Other advantages of sclerotherapy will be discussed in Chapter 14.

The successful development and use of sclerosing agents for varicose veins naturally led to an extension of this therapy for sclerosing purposes elsewhere in the body. A description of the individual sclerosing agents developed and successfully used up to the present time follows:

Sodium Morrhuate

Originally the name *morrhuic acid* was given by Gautier and Mourges (12) to a ntirogenous putrefaction product, hydroxydihydrophyridine butyric acid ($C_9H_{13}NO_3$) found in rotted cod-liver oil. The name, sodium morrhuate, was originally used as an elegant synonym for cod-liver oil extract prepared for intravenous injection by the methods devised by Ghosh (13) or Cutting (14).

Table 1

SOLUTIONS USED IN SCLEROTHERAPY

Order of Increasing Sclerotic Power

	Solution	Classification	Amount Injected	Untoward Reactions	Indication
1	Dextrose 25-50%	Organic	2-20 c.c.	None	Latent phlebitis
2	Invert Sugar 60%	Organic	2-20 c.c.	Cramp only occasionally	Phlebitis and routinely as first injection
3	Sodium Chloride 20-30%	Dehydrant	5-20 c.c.	Cramp	Dilated venules for smooth thrombosis
4	Dextrose and NaCl	Mixed Dehydrant	5-20 c.c.	Cramp	Where smooth cosmetic result is desired in varicose veins
5	Sylnasol 5% & 10%	Soap	2-5 c.c.	Renal colic	Varicose veins
6	Aethoxysclerol	Synthetic, Alcohol base	1-4 c.c.	None	Varicose veins, venules
7	Scleremo	Chromate	1-5 c.c.	None	Varicose veins
8	Variglobin 1%, 3%, 5% & 10%	$KI\text{-}I_2$	1-3 c.c.	None	Varicose veins
9	Sodium Morrhuate	Soap	2-10 c.c.	Dermatitis	Varicose veins
10	Momoethanolamine Oleate (Monolate)	Soap	1-3 c.c.	None	Varicose veins, resistant veins
11	Soricin 2% & 3½%	Soap	2-5 c.c.	Local burning	Routine and large veins
12	Ipotole	Soap	1-10 c.c.	None	Routine and large saphenous veins
13	Etalate	Soap	1-10 c.c.	None	Routine and large saphenous veins
14	Sotradecol 1% & 3% (Trombovar) European product	Synthetic	1-5 c.c.	Pigmentation, fever occasionally	Routine — most veins
15	Morrhu-Quin	Mixture	No longer used		
16	Koleo-Quinine	Mixture	No longer used		
17	Quinine and Urethane	Organic	1-3 c.c.	Cinchonism, Pigmentation	Varicose veins, resistant veins
18	Sodium Salicylate 30-40%	Dehydrant	1-3 c.c.	Intense cramp	Resistant veins
19	Bichloride of Mercury 1%	Heavy Metal	½-1 c.c.	Pain, hydragyria	Rarely used except in stubborn sclerotic varicose veins

Sodium morrhuate itself is a yellow, fishy smelling powder that has a greasy soapy feel. It dissolves in water to make a light yellow solution that lathers like soap on agitation. This mixture is unstable on standing if exposed to air. In about a week of such exposure it forms a fine white cloudy precipitate. The originators who prepared this solution for the treatment of tuberculosis observed that even in sterile amber bottles tightly sealed for a week deterioration took place.

In powder form it does not hold up well at all. In a few days at best a dark insoluble product forms. Obviously a solution is a better method of preserving this agent and some means of preventing oxidation had to be developed.

Sodium morrhuate is far from being a simple solution. It has a very complicated structure containing over 90 unsaturated fatty acids, some of which have not yet been identified. A partial list of these fatty acids includes: myristic, palmitic, palmitoleic, stearic, oleic, eruchic, therapic, and others too numerous to mention. *Bills** isolated over 90 with more to go. Most of these are unsaturated and comparatively unstable. Furthermore, the degree of unsaturation of a particular sample of oil depends upon the proportions of unsaturated acids present, and varies with each batch tested. The variations in oil depend upon other factors beyond our control such as the feeding ground of the fish, the season of the year, and the sexual differences. In spite of these fluctuations in composition, when the product is made in the standard fashion, the therapeutic responses are uniform enough to warrant retention as a routine sclerosing agent.

I have used this reagent over a period of fifty years and find that its manufacture is being constantly improved. For years it has been made with the addition of 2% benzyl alcohol which acts as an antiseptic as well as a local anesthetic. The basic powder is now more refined than in previous years, and the solutions obtained from it are obviously better filtered by using improved modern micropore filters.

The color of the improved sodium morrhuate solution is much paler, almost colorless, when compared with the older solutions which were in various shades of amber. Care must be observed in using it, however, that the plunger of the syringe does not get stuck to the barrel. The older solution was much more soapy and less apt to cause sticking. It is advisable, with the newer preparations, to use the solutions immediately after filling the syringe. However, it has an advantage in that cloudiness in the ampule or vial is much less apt to occur on standing.

---

* Mead Johnson & Co. chemist

The dosage of sodium morrhuate in 5% solution varies from ½ to 5 c.c. Only occasionally have I used 8 c.c. in one dose. The average injection is 2 c.c. Various factors have to be evaluated in deciding how much to inject for each vein.

This reagent and others equally potent should not be employed as a first injection. Instead, one must use a safe medication for varicose veins. This should be a solution of salt or sugar or a mixture of both. These will now be described (see Table 1).

Salt and Sugar

Sugar solutions comprise the blandest type of sclerosing agents that are still employed. An early form was invert sugar 60% used by Kausch of Germany, 1917. This is a dark brown viscous solution containing invertose dissolved in water. It was formerly used for small veins and as a mild sclerosant to start a case of varicose veins. Since invert sugar may have a varying amount of glucose and levulose, and because of its syrupy character, it is no longer in common use. However, it is still a good mild sclerosing agent and may be employed as such. Dextrose, the mildest of the sugar reagents, can be used in concentrations up to 50%. It is valuable in 25% strength as a provocative first injection. It may activate a phlebitic condition to a mild degree but in the average varicose vein it will have little or no effect. As noted in Table 1, in large amounts (10 to 20 c.c.), it may produce slight cramping. It should not produce necrosis unless significant amounts of the 50% concentration escape into delicate tissues with poor circulation.

Sodium chloride in 0.9% dilution is physiologic and can be injected almost anywhere in the body. When used in 15% to 30% concentrations it becomes a potent sclerosing agent. Solutions of 18% to 30% are extremely useful for capillaries and small venule injection.

When dextrose and sodium chloride are combined, the potency of the mixture as a sclerosing liquid is increased. The combination is then useful as a general sclerosing preparation for routine use in varicose veins. Originally made by combining invert sugar, 30%, with sodium chloride, 10%, under the trade name of *Varisol**, the mixture was completed by the addition of phenylethyl alcohol 1% and propylene glycol 10%. This was a stable mixture manufactured in a special way** to enhance its stability. (Table 1) The physician using these reagents may make his own preparations along these lines. It is a comparatively simple procedure to mix salt and sugar solutions together because it is now

---

* Abbott & Co.

** In ampules containing inert gases.

possible to get sterile vials of both reagents and to combine them in the desired ratio prior to the actual injection.

Sylnasol

Sylnasol, 5% and 10%, aqueous solution was manufactured from the oil of psyllium seeds and converted into a liquid soap by saponification. It is not made in the United States at the present time but is obtainable elsewhere.

Sylnasol had a wide range of usefulness as a mild sclerosing agent in varicose veins, hernia, and low back therapy. An occasional peculiar side effect of this medication in varicose veins was the production of a transient renal colic upon injection of 2 to 5 c.c. in medium size or large veins of the leg or thigh. This was best explained by the probable backing up or reflux of the solution into the kidney through the renal vein which ordinarily has no valve. After a few minutes, the pain always disappeared without any remaining symptoms.

Soricin

Soricin 2% and 3½%, a liquid soap made from castor oil was another sodium salt preparation which had a more irritating action in varicose veins than Sylnasol. Its place on the table of varicose vein irritants (Table 1) was number 11, indicating its position in sclerotic power. It was useful as a routine solution in the large veins of the thigh.

Ipotole

Ipotole was a saponified solution of purified olive oil made into a sclerosing agent. This followed my report in 1933 (15) where I described the use of sodium oleate 5% experimentally for varicose veins.

Subsequently, this oleate solution was manufactured as potassium oleate 5% and called Ipotole. Its use was attended by firm sclerosis of varicose veins. This product led the way to other soapy medications.

Morrhu-quin and Koleo-quinine

Morrhu-quin and Koleo-quinine were combinations of fatty acid solutions with quinine. These mixtures enhanced the action of sodium morrhuate by the addition of a potent sclerosing agent, quinine. They had sclerosing power of a high order and are interesting in the evolution of today's synthetic fatty acid preparations. They are rarely used today. Aside from the historical interest, their obsolescence is not to be deplored because they were unscientific and unnecessarily cumbersome.

Monolate and Etalate

Monolate and Etalate were the first synthetic oleates to be produced in the evolving chain of sclerosing agents. Chemically, they are monoethanolamine oleate and ethylenamine oleate. They are oleate salts where the sodium or potassium ions are replaced by organic synthetic radicals. Strictly speaking they are only partially synthetic because the oleate radical is prepared from olive oil which is a natural product. These solutions were very effective sclerosing agents with definite formulae, but caused occasional allergic reactions due to traces of protein in the parent olive oil which were not eliminated in the purification process. Monolate is still in use outside of the United States.

Sodium Salicylate

Before turning to the latest group of synthetic preparations it is necessary to review several older solutions which are still available. Sodium salicylate 12% to 60% has been in use for over fifty years as a powerful sclerosing solution. While it is very effective as an endothelial irritant, its use is accompanied by intense cramping and an undesirable necrotic action if inadvertently injected perivascularly. It can be used with Procaine or Xylocaine in the formula to subdue the cramping. There are occasional instances when I still resort to this powerful solution but use it with great circumspection.

Quinine and Urethane

Quinine and urethane is one of the oldest solutions that was used for varicose veins and is still occasionally employed. It is available in 2 c.c. ampules containing:

Quinine Hydrochloride	0.26 Gms.
Urethane	0.13 Gms.
Distilled Water – to equal	2 c.c.

It is one of the most potent sclerosing agents but does not fit into modern sclerotherapy for varicose veins because of the undesirable side effects of tinnitus and dizziness. However, it is very useful for stubborn veins where no more than 2 c.c. of this solution is required. As an addition to our armamentarium it has value within its limits.

Metals

Among the metallic solutions still available is bichloride of mercury 1%. This is rarely, almost never, used. It is a toxic heavy metal solution and is the most potent corrosive preparation for varicose veins that is obtainable. It cannot be used in more than 1 c.c. quantities because of its mercurial content. When it is needed for special occasions, it can be depended upon to close a very stubborn, thickly walled calcified vein (Table 1).

Scleremo

Scleremo is a preparation containing glycerine chromate 1.11% which is classified with the metallic salts and is used in 1 to 5 c.c. amounts for routine sclerotherapy of varicose veins. I have never seen any allergy resulting from this preparation. It is used in France extensively for varicose veins and hemorrhoids.

Variglobin

Variglobin for varicose veins was formerly available in varying strengths from ½ to 12%.* This is a chemical combination copied from Lugol's solution which has been in general medical use orally for over a hundred years. However, instead of the sodium iodide ingredient of Lugol's solution, this mixture contains potassium iodide which is better tolerated for intravenous use. The potassium iodide and iodine are in a loose chemical combination with a continuously reversible equilibrium so that there is always some free iodine in the mixture in ionic form. This preparation has been and still is extensively used in Europe for the routine treatment of varicose veins. It has a voluminous bibliography and has been extensively tested and reported upon for twenty years. My studies, 1961 to 1966,** corroborated these findings. There were practically no allergic manifestations.

Sotradecol

Sotradecol is the leading sclerosing agent for general use in all types of varicose veins as mentioned earlier in this chapter. Its European counterpart, with the same chemical formula, is called Trombovar, and is also the leading medication for sclerosing purposes in Europe.

Sotradecol is a clear, colorless solution with a dependable, constant formulation that produces predictable uniform results in varicose vein therapy. The 1% dilution is suitable for smaller veins while the 3% form will sclerose all of the larger veins if used properly. Sometimes the injection of this material in susceptible individuals is followed by pigmentation of the skin. This occurs more often with the higher concentration of 3% than with the weaker solution. This will be taken up in more detail in the chapter on cosmetic aspects (Chapter 14). Allergy is infrequent following its use.

Aethoxysklerol

Aethoxysklerol is also a totally synthesized development containing ethyl alcohol in its formulation. The concentration of alcohol, while only 5%, makes a marked difference in the action of the sclerosing chemical, hydroxypolyaethoxydodecan. Marketed in Europe as Aethoxysklerol, it is available in four strengths: 0.5%, 1%, 2% and 3%. The 2 and 3% strengths are suitable for routine varicose vein therapy. The 1 and 0.5% strengths are useful in the treatment of fine venules, capillaries, and blotchy areas. These discolorations are difficult to classify from a dermatological point of view. The virtue of the 0.5% solution is that it is practically slough proof and may be injected subcutaneously and perivascularly for its effect on capillary enlargements and discolored, blemished areas. The 3% solution, if used in amounts above 1 or 2 c.c.,

* Recently solutions of 20% have been used.

** Two statistical series of clinical testing submitted to the FDA.

produces varying amounts of pain momentarily. While the dilute solution is placed number 6 on the scale of sclerosing agents, this applies only to the 0.5% and the 1%. When used in 3 c.c. quantities of the 3% strength, it can be more properly classified with Sotradecol as one of the strongest sclerosing agents in Table 1.*

These are the solutions past and present used for sclerotherapy in varicose veins. It is important to record them because medical preferences vary from time to time, and while new ones are being formulated, some of the older preparations may be revived. As stated previously, there can never be too many sclerosing solutions because no two cases are exactly alike in their requirements. Furthermore, while FDA restrictions preclude the use of some solutions in this country, they are being employed in countries that have different regulations.

In the succeeding chapters it will be shown that due to sensitivities, allergies, phlebitis, and anatomical differences the treatment, and with it the solutions, will vary from one case to another. Without such a diversity of injectibles, it might not be possible to effectively and safely treat all the patients who present themselves.

*Recently aqueous solutions up to 4% have been developed for varicose veins.

Chapter 4

▪ STANDARD TECHNIQUE FOR INJECTION TREATMENT OF VARICOSE VEINS

This technique is suitable for the novice as well as the experienced physician. It is used whenever the operator or patient prefers a leisurely approach to this therapy. It is also employed for teaching programs so that the pupil can more readily grasp the significance of the step by step approach to the finished technique.

Before describing the actual injection treatments I must point out that there is a bewildering variety of varicose vein patterns, no two of which are exactly alike. The veins involved are all part of the saphenous system described in Chapter 1. They include the great saphenous veins, the lesser saphenous group, and the communicating veins, also known as the muscular perforators. Aside from rare arteriovenous shunts there are no other types of varicose veins to consider. We are not including telangiectasia (spider veins) in this discussion as their treatment will be described separately in Chapter 13.

Stand-up Method versus Empty-Vein Techniques

We must also deal with the differences between the stand-up method and empty-vein techniques.

I do not find it realistic to perform the exacting work of varicose vein sclerotherapy without at some point, treating the patient in the upright position. On the other hand, there are those who have become so impressed with empty-vein techniques, that they attempt to use them almost exclusively. Between these two views there is a diversity of opinions regarding the degree to which individual doctors favor either one technique or a combination of both. The technique in the upright position will be described next while more rapid methods and empty-vein techniques will follow (Chapter 5).

Order of Injections

The doctor is comfortably seated in front of the treatment table. The patient stands on top of the treatment table, facing the doctor, whose eyes are on a level with the knee area (Fig. 3). In this position it is convenient to inject from the groins down to the feet with perhaps standing up to reach the highest point of the great saphenous system adjoining the groin.

The order of injections has always been a mystifying problem for the neophyte who must often make quick decisions. A set of principles that will guide the beginner is as follows (see Fig. 8):

1. Start in a safe area in the mid-leg to minimize reactions;
2. Inject from above down except when closing the great saphenous vein which requires special handling;
3. In cases that are complicated by phlebitis, it will be necessary to modify the treatment (see Phlebitis, Chapter 7);
4. Treat the great saphenous vein as soon as the necessary preliminary veins are closed;
5. Treat the ankle and foot area last.

These rules are elastic and are varied to suit the case.

The First Injection.

This should always be the mildest irritant available. For instance, we can use ½ c.c. to 1 c.c. of 50% dextrose or 60% invert sugar solution (Table 1).

The location is always on the leg. A medium-size varicosity in the mid-leg region is chosen in order to study the reaction to the sclerosing solution. Sometimes a latent phlebitis will be activated by the first injection. The reaction to watch for may start within three to five hours and consists of an area of tenderness or thrombosis which can be seen or felt if the patient remains in the office. Otherwise, it will be reported by the patient and confirmed by the doctor on the next office visit.

Subsequent Injections

The operator must now plan his treatment schedule. He must decide whether to treat his patient once or twice a week. The more conservative plan will be for a series of weekly injections requiring two to three months to complete an advanced case.

If the schedule is on a weekly basis, the second visit can consist of one or two injections, depending upon the results of the test injection.

If there was no reaction or just a minimal result, the operator may proceed with ½ to 1 c.c. of sodium morrhuate as the second injection. This, again, should be in the mid- or upper-leg area, avoiding at this time large varicosities, if possible.

Where the condition is bilateral, each leg may be treated in this fashion or one leg may be treated first and the reaction noted several hours later before doing the other leg. This will give the operator an opportunity to study the patients' reaction to the medication. A pronounced swelling of the vein wall with accompanying redness calls for moderation in treatment. This can be achieved by reducing the dosage by half.

After each injection a sterile ball, approximately three quarters to one inch in diameter, made of gauze preferably or cotton, is placed over the vein, and strapped down with one-inch strips of adhesive. Some technicians use additional compression (see compression sclerotherapy, Chapter 5). This may consist of foam rubber sheeting and gauze bandage, or various types of elastic bandaging. Rubber moulds* made in Europe are also used.

The injections are usually continued on a weekly basis. There is another rule here which will aid in determining the strength and amount of sclerosing solution. This is to always use the mildest sclerosing agent that will produce satisfactory closure of the vein. There is no advantage in exceeding this dosage.

To apply this important rule, the operator must know the order of increasing power of the various sclerosing reagents. Table 1 grades these solutions both past and present by listing them in such an order. The wide variety and number of sclerosing agents should be appreciated because there are still others that have been omitted for clarity.

Some of these solutions are only of historic interest, but I feel they must all be retained in our armamentarium because there can never be an overabundance of sclerosing agents.

A good technician can only do better work with such a large reserve of solutions. Each individual patient may be a special problem and some can only be treated with just one of these agents if he happens to be allergic to all the rest.

The ideal reaction is a firm, small diameter thrombosis without excessive tenderness. With experience, the proper dosage can be gauged accurately enough to produce this. Minimal thrombosis without tenderness can be achieved without empty-vein technique after the operator learns to gauge the sclerosing dosage accurately.

---

* Preformed specially shaped rubber forms are available from European sources.

The great saphenous vein in the thigh is next in order of attack (Fig. 8). If this important vein does not show on the surface, it should be located and identified by palpation, percussion, or both. In percussing the saphenous vein, the operator or his assistant taps a visible vein segment on the leg with one hand while one or the other palpates for the main trunk on the internal thigh with the other hand. Once located, it may readily be injected by an empty-vein technique, if desired (see Chapter 5).

Referring again to Fig. 8, it will be noted that tributaries of the internal saphenous are next injected. Working from above down, the veins are treated in orderly progression. The varicosities around the ankle and dorsum of the foot are done last.

After the internal saphenous and its branches are completed, the lesser saphenous system is attacked. The same general rules apply. Working from above down, the main trunk and its tributaries are sclerosed. This system will also contribute branches to the ankle in the lateral malleolus area and dorsum of the foot. All of this must be carefully injected.

Perforator veins, which penetrate below the fascia, must be injected next for a complete result if they have not been treated already. This may be accomplished by injecting the branches connected with the perforator vein, or carefully injecting the perforator vein itself, to get satisfactory closure. An empty-vein technique for perforator veins is described in Chapter 5.

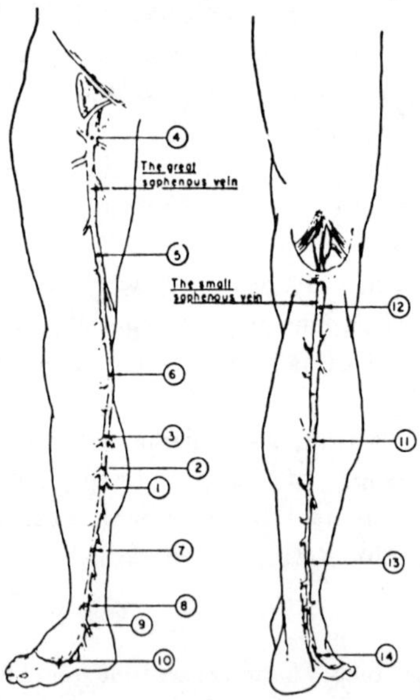

Figure 8. Order of injection.

As one proceeds with the weekly schedule and in the absence of allergy or phlebitis, a gradual increase in the strength of the sclerosing solutions is needed. Thus, if the second treatment has been ½ to 1 c.c. of sodium morrhuate, the third could well be 2 c.c. of the same reagent, or the more potent sotradecol can be started. Two or three treatments can be given on the third visit. In the absence of marked reaction, once the dosage of 2 c.c. sotradecol has been reached, three or four treatments may be given at one sitting. If a total of 4 to 6 c.c. of sclerosing solution is given one week, this amount may be increased to 8 c.c. the following week. These amounts, of course, are the totals of several injections and do not indicate one large treatment. The dosages are subject to the operator's judgement and experience.

The ankle and dorsum of the foot is the point of greatest venous pressure and stagnation in cases of varicose veins. In addition, there is very little subcutaneous tissue present. These tissues cannot tolerate the same degree of irritation as those higher up on the leg. Consequently, the injections must be in much smaller amounts and less potent in sclerotic power, otherwise sloughing may develop, even with well-placed injections.

One must be on the alert for allergy in this weekly method of injection treatments. A clue may often be given by the appearance of one or two local or distant wheals following treatment. This is an indication of a possible allergic manifestation which may suddenly show at the next session. In the event of such a warning signal it is urgent that the operator switch to another type of sclerosing solution, bearing in mind that various members of the fatty acid group may exhibit cross-sensitivities. Therefore, if one member of this group, such as sodium morrhuate, reacts with a few wheals, it is sometimes advisable to discontinue the entire fatty-acid group, and use a sclerosing agent from a different family.

Another reaction to be on guard for is the phlebitic one. This may arise from a latent covert phlebitis lurking in the veins, and a flare-up may result at any point in the early phases of the treatment. Some indication of latent phlebitis may be obtained with the first provocative test injection. Whereas a normal vein will not react to the weak first sugar test (½ c.c. glucose or invert sugar), in the case of latent phlebitis, a slight to moderate tender perivenous induration may develop within several hours. This calls for caution in succeeding treatments to avoid a violent flare-up. For instance, a slight inflammatory result to the test injection should be followed by 2 c.c. of the sugar or other weak solution on the next occasion. If there is no reaction, the third dose could then be 1 or 2 c.c. of sodium morrhuate. It is important to understand that even a slight inflammatory result protects the patient against marked flare-up reactions. While we don't know the exact explanation for this, we can conjecture that immunity is developing to the phlebitic process because subsequent injections are usually well borne without inflammatory responses.

This schedule is followed until all the varicosities are sclerosed.

Resume of Standard Injection Treatment

While I don't often find this older method of injecting varicose veins useful in my practice, I have carefully described it for important reasons. It is a good way for the novice to learn injection therapy of varicose veins. It has applicability for all levels of competence where slow and minutely controlled treatment is indicated. It is a sound basis for understanding the rationale and technique of the newer rapid method and empty-vein techniques.

The diverse variety of cases that present themselves has been indicated. The order of injections has been listed but it must be emphasized that this is subject to wide differences in individual cases and the doctor must adapt this treatment to fit the case. For instance, if the patient shows a large saphenous with a great many leg branches, it becomes a matter of clinical judgment when to sclerose the main vein. If the vein is closed too soon, it may not be possible to locate and treat all the branches because they may almost disappear with effective large vein closure.

On the other hand, with only a few large leg branches it is usually advisable to close the large saphenous first, because there will be no problem in finding and treating the lower branches.

Special indications connected with the degree of phlebitis, skin complications, and other conditions will influence the order of injections.

The ideal reaction has been described. It is not often realized, but the greater judgment and skill the operator possesses, the closer he will come to achieving such symptom-free results. A knowledge of the order of increasing power of sclerosing solutions is needed for competence. The perforator veins are in a special category and are dealt with after the saphenous veins have been treated in most cases.

The ankle area, which is a delicate part of the limb, must be treated with respect. Lastly, allergic and phlebitic reactions which occur more frequently with this slower method, must be understood in order to manage them properly.

I favor the rapid method of sclerotherapy in most cases because of its outstanding advantages as will be described in the following chapter.

Chapter 5

▪ AUTHOR'S RAPID METHOD AND COMPRESSION SCLEROTHERAPY

This technique was developed through necessity. Patients coming from a long distance found it impossible to embark on a treatment program lasting for weeks or months. By modifying my original standard weekly treatment schedule (Chapter 4), the average case was condensed into three days.

The three day program in many cases rapidly became a standard procedure. Occasionally, it was expedient to concentrate this treatment further into a 24 hour program which made injection treatment even faster than surgery. Occasionally patients exhibiting active phlebitis required an additional fourth or a fifth day of treatment. It was rare to find a patient who could not be finished within a two week period of treatment.

What was extremely gratifying was to find a treatment regimen, originally designed for patients traveling from distant areas, so strikingly successful that it became standard procedure for all cases. This unexpected development might not have arisen so readily under ordinary circumstances of medical practice.

I was at first apprehensive about developing this treatment method because of four possible complications. These were pain, allergy, phlebitis, and embolism.

It was soon apparent that any pain produced by this condensed treatment schedule was no greater than that following the regular weekly injections. Thus, with a series of four injections given at weekly intervals, each one might produce separate inflammatory responses. The similar treatments rendered consecutively on the same day produced diminishing reactions or even no reactions after the first one.

While we do not understand completely the nature of the responses involved, it is clear that multiple treatments do not increase the painful effects of varicose vein injections.

Allergic reactions are also considerably reduced in number and degree with this rapid method of treatment. If the patient has not been previously sensitized to the injection material, multiple treatments tend to reduce allergic responses. However, the first injection possibly containing allergenic substances must be watched very closely for a possible reaction. If there is none, the probability of inducing further atopic responses is very small because it takes approximately one week's time for antibodies to develop and produce allergic responses. If the injections are given rapidly within this time span, there should be no such manifestation.

Immediate constitutional reaction is a possibility here as with the standard treatment method, but usually only with the early injections of the series. This should be guarded against with the history and careful observation. Sometimes skin rashes will appear as a warning signal of impending allergy.

When it comes to phlebitic reactions we are again fortunate that this concentrated method yields less of these responses than with the older weekly technique. I have found that overwhelming the body's responses makes the development of phlebitis a far less frequent occurrence. Whatever the nature of phlebitis complicating varicose veins is, it takes time for a phlebitic reaction to develop. By giving injections closely spaced, there is also no time available to build up a phlebitic reaction. During this reaction-free time period the important large veins in the varicose system can be effectively sclerosed without such reaction.

Up to the present, the nature of superficial phlebitis, especially in varicose veins, is still not clear. Nevertheless, the thrombotic responses to sclerotherapy and their control have been studied and clarified. This rapid method is ideal for the ordinary case of varicose veins even when accompanied by mild to moderate phlebitis.

There are individuals who exhibit acute flare-ups of phlebitis, where I do not advocate an immediate attack on the varicose condition. Due to the potential for dangerous reactions, one should allow additional time for evaluating these cases before attempting injection treatment. This will be described in greater detail (Chapter 7).

Looking back over an experience of fifty years, I agree with other observers (16) that the fear of embolism following injection treatment of varicose veins is largely unfounded. In my experience it has occurred only *five times* in many thousands of injections. The frequency of this complication is no greater with rapid technique than with the old, slower method of treatment. Furthermore, it becomes less frequent with the operators increasing experience.

I feel that the emphasis on compression will further reduce this complication. I also caution the patient against vigorous exercise with rapid treatment, limiting physical activity to mild forms like walking or swimming. More strenuous sports, such as tennis or even golf, are not permitted for three weeks following treatment. Horseback riding is forbidden for two months.*

There is a greater need for empty-vein techniques with the rapid method, to prevent recanalization. With the old slower method, any vein that doesn't close, or starts to recanalize, can be reinjected during the following weeks of treatment. After concentrated treatment, the operator must observe special precautions because there is less time to make corrections. The technique described below calls for inspecting each group of injections at the end of each session, with a final examination at the close of each day.

Recanalization Versus New Varicose Vein Formation

There is controversy whether varicosities appearing after a variable period of time following sclerotherapy are due to recanalization of injected veins or a new growth of varicosities. It has been difficult to differentiate between these two kinds of development.

Some observers insist that all *recurrences* are due to ineffective treatment, mainly in the bandaging. This permits the venous pressure to dissect and separate the thromboses into layers, and ultimately reproduce the vascular channels and recurrent varicose veins. With competent treatment and pressure bandaging, this should not happen. It is particularly prone to appear at the sapheno-femoral junction at the fossa ovalis and the entrances to the series of perforator veins in the leg and thigh.

Other observers believe that many of the new varicosities following a course of veno-therapy are actually new formations arising from satellite veins, vena comites, or normal veins that now grow in response to the trauma of the vascular tree by injection treatment.

I have observed many times in patients who develop a regrowth of varicose veins that definite cordlike evidences of firmly thrombosed vein segments lie parallel to clearly newly developed varicosities. The repeated finding of both old and new varicosities, lying side by side to each other, can have no explanation other than new vein formation.

While attempts have been made by phlebography to study the ultimate fate of injected veins, there is as yet no satisfactory technique to settle this dispute other than the clinical observations I have described. As discussed in the section on chronicity of veins (Chapter 11), even after heroic surgery in competent hands has been completed for the removal of varicose veins and there is absolutely no possibility of recanalization, there are still numerous cases exhibiting the development of an entirely new saphenous and perforator vein system. In my studies (17), they took 5 to 20 years to develop. There has

* Some observers do not limit physical activity at all. More statistical studies are needed.

been no long-term acceptable and confirmed statistical series that has refuted this evidence. More research is needed in this area.

There are two general methods of injecting varicosities using the rapid technique and also two types of pressure bandaging. These will be discussed before outlining the actual technique.

Full Vein Techniques (Upright Positions)

Full vein technique cannot be discarded because many, female patients especially, present themselves for treatment because of cosmetic reasons. Small varicosities, venules of various sizes, small vein clusters around the ankle and foot, in addition to other subcutaneous varicosities elsewhere on the limb, require the standing position for proper injection treatment.

I have found that an experienced operator working on the usual small to medium-sized varicosities can secure sclerosis with a minimum of thrombosis, if the proper dosage of sclerosing agent is used. This can be aided by various maneuvers to localize the solution while keeping the vein as flat as possible. Using the fingers properly, this can be achieved while the patient is standing or, sometimes, sitting. When properly performed, the resulting thrombus is equivalent to that produced by the average empty-vein method.

There is no purpose in emptying these small blood vessels because, when empty, they cannot be located and treated effectively, In my experience, many women requesting treatment for varicose veins do not require therapy for the great saphenous vein in the thigh or communicating veins in the extremity. They present themselves for cosmetic reasons and deserve treatment on that basis.

Empty-Vein Techniques

This is not a new concept in sclerotherapy. It was recognized at the outset when attempts were made to localize the action of the sclerosing solution by various means such as occluders, tourniquets, and special clamps. Operators quickly learned that their fingers could isolate a vein segment, and by stroking, partially empty the vein of its blood, enhancing the action of the sclerosing fluid as noted above.

The next step was the introduction of phlebotomy for the great saphenous vein in the thigh in an attempt to empty this large vessel while the patient remained erect. With the valves above permitting a partial reflux of blood, it was possible to decrease the volume of this large trunk to a point where injection treatment was more efficient. This was not a true empty-vein technique

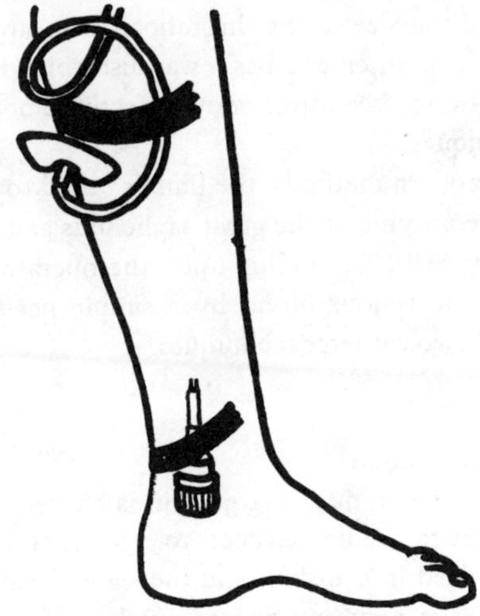

Figure 9. Upper-butterfly needle in place. Lower-Catheter needle in place; hub attached for mobility of leg.

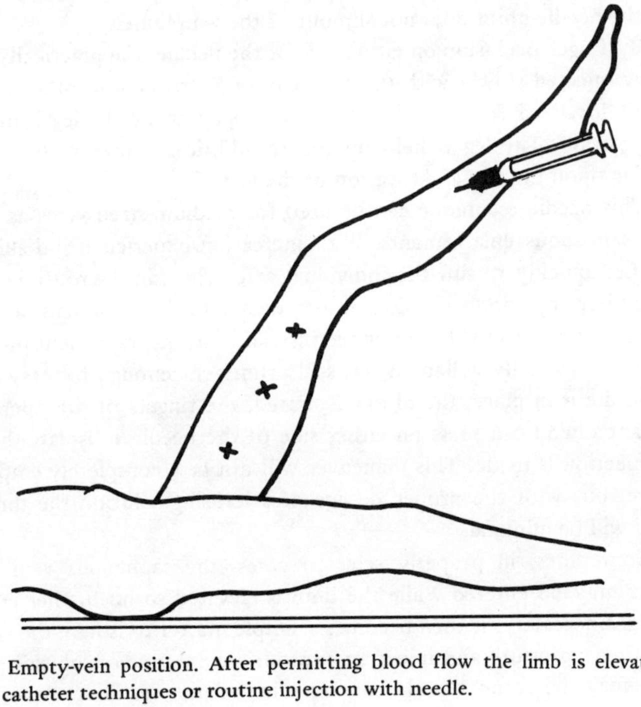

Figure 10. Empty-vein position. After permitting blood flow the limb is elevated for injection by catheter techniques or routine injection with needle.

although it reduced the size of the thrombosis. The large volume of blood that had to be drained into an emesis basin was disturbing to many patients. Treatment remained static for years until more effective blood drainage was achieved by improved techniques.

In all of the modern methods, the limb is raised to a 45 or 90 degree angle for more efficient emptying of the great saphenous and perforator vein systems (see Fig. 9 and Fig. 10). Depending upon the operator's choice and training, he may withdraw the venous blood by a simple needle technique or, if preferred, by either of two catheter techniques.

Individual Needle Technique

With this needle technique, a large vein is chosen with the patient sitting. Using a 19 to 22 gauge needle attached to a 5 c.c. syringe, the vein is entered, the needle immobilized in the skin, and the leg is elevated to a 45 degree angle cautiously. The vein is now emptied as much as possible by aspiration after which another syringe containing Sotradecol 3% is substituted for the first syringe. Great care must be observed throughout the whole procedure to insure that the needle point does not slip out of the vein lumen.

By finger occlusion on either side of the needle, the practically empty vein is now injected slowly with 0.5 to 1 c.c. of Sotradecol or other solution. This is kept localized for one minute by the fingers while the leg is maintained in this position. The leg is held up for an additional three to four minutes depending upon the size and location of the vein.

This needle technique can be used for medium-sized veins as well as huge great saphenous enlargements. With increasing experience and skill, it can be modified quickly to suit the individual case. Thus, in the routine management of stand-up injections, the doctor may decide to sit the patient down and treat a bulging vein with the leg extended instead of in the dependent position. Here, the vein is partially collapsed but still prominent enough for easy entry. After the needle is in place, the blood aspirated, the fingers of the operator's or his assistant's hand can press on either side of the needle to isolate the vein while the injection is made. This maneuver will not be a completely empty-vein procedure, but with the proper dosage of sclerosing solution the thrombus produced will be minimal.

Sometimes, in properly selected cases, the saphenous vein or its large trunks may be entered while the limb is elevated so no further movement of the leg is necessary. It then becomes a simple matter to isolate the vein segment with finger pressure and inject an appropriate amount of solution. In this case there may be some blood remaining in a large segment; nevertheless, the resulting thrombus will be considerably reduced and should heal properly with sufficient, extended compression time.

Another possibility occurs when large, bulging varicosities, often connected with perforator veins, present themselves on the calf of the leg. Here I have obtained good sclerosis with small thrombi by piercing the vein with the patient in the prone position and making the injection after the knee is bent to a 90 degree angle.

The amount of sclerosing fluid used in all of these empty or partially empty-vein techniques will vary in each case. A good general rule is that whenever the venous stream is slowed, or the blood volume in the treated vein is reduced by any technique, a corresponding decrease in sclerosing power is called for. In fact, even in the standing position, injections around the foot and ankle should be reduced in potency because here the venous stream is often at its slowest.

Catheter Techniques

I began the use of catheters for empty-vein techniques in 1975 to prevent the errors which threatened occasionally by needles slipping out of the vein during limb movements such as extension and elevation. Two types of catheter needles are in use. They are the butterfly catheter needle and the stylet type catheter needle. These have been mentioned in Chapter 2, but now the details of their use will be described.

The butterfly type needle (Figs. 1, 9) resembles a butterfly, the wings of which can be immobilized with a narrow strip of adhesive after the veins has been punctured. As in the previous procedure for treating the great saphenous vein, the needle is inserted and strapped into position with the patient sitting on the operating table. Removal of the small cap at the end of the plastic catheter will permit blood flow which can be seen and collected in a basin. The limb can now be raised to a 45 degree angle (Fig. 10) and by the use of a 10 to 20 c.c. syringe, blood can be withdrawn until the vein is empty. Then, the appropriate sclerosing solution in the syringe is attached to the plastic catheter and is slowly injected while the proximal and distal segments of the vein are compressed.

The butterfly needle is now removed and a gauze sponge placed over the skin puncture which is strapped into position firmly by adhesive strips. The limb is kept elevated from three to five minutes and then lowered. This method, while efficient, still leaves 0.25 c.c. of blood in the vein being treated. This comes from the catheter itself and can be practically eliminated if the plastic tube is shortened and a special adapter attached to it for the purpose of receiving the tip of the syringe. However, the few drops of blood left behind in a large saphenous vein does not alter appreciably the sclerosing action of the solution used or the size of the thrombus in the treated vein. This method has given good results with small or no thrombi.

The stylet type catheter needles are on a different order and permit ambulation of the patient after they are inserted into the vein. They were originally developed for routine use in hospitals for intravenous instillations and are still used there. They are valuable for empty vein techniques in the treatment of varicose veins and are available in several sizes (Fig. 2).

To understand their use in varicose veins, a brief description of the needle assembly is necessary. It is composed of three parts:

1) The flexible plastic catheter on a standard hub that can receive a hypodermic syringe tip;

2) A metal catheter needle which fits inside the plastic catheter so that its tip protrudes slightly enabling the operator to inject and place the needle combination inside the vein; and,

3) A plastic stylet attached to another hub which screws into the catheter hub.

The needle assembly is inserted into the vein with the patient standing or sitting. The hub, with attached plastic catheter, is advanced into the vein by a twisting motion usually, until it can go no further, sometimes up to the skin surface.

It is then strapped down with a narrow band of adhesive, after which the needle is removed from the flexible catheter that remains in the vein (Fig. 9). Some blood flow occurs at this point which is effectively checked by insertion of the plastic solid stylet through the hub into the flexible catheter. The stylet is now tightened on the catheter hub, thereby permitting motion of the limb without bleeding or catheter displacement. It is now possible to have the patient walk to an operating table where he will lie down, elevate his leg, and receive the sclerosing injection after removal of the plastic stylet. Any vein in the leg or thigh may be emptied of blood and treated in this fashion, if desired (Fig. 10). The reaction obtained will be minimal in size and tenderness, thereby improving the results.

Perforator Technique

Incompetent perforator veins should be sought at the beginning of each case. Mention has been made that one-third of the patients in my experience exhibit only superficial varicosities without any large vein involvement. Of the remaining two-thirds, some have incompetence at the sapheno-femoral junction, some show incompetent perforator veins while the rest have both types to a variable degree. All three types require treatment for effective results.

The detection of incompetent perforator veins usually is a simple matter. With the patient standing, the Trendelenberg tests, especially with a negative reaction, will give some indication of their existence. They are often visible in advanced cases and can be palpated in their early phases as varices arising from openings in the fascial and muscular layers beneath the surface of the leg or thigh. Sherman (18), who made an extensive study of the perforator vein system, described them accurately and with great detail in his report. He was of the opinion that the thorough excision of these veins, when dilated, was imperative.

Fegan (19) locates perforator veins by inspecting and marking the extremity with the patient erect, which is followed by papation of the elevated leg with the patient lying down. Weaknesses or orifices in the fascia are revealed by palpation, and he states that fingers may be introduced into each orifice and the skin marked appropriately. He finds that in many of his patients one fascial orifice may control the filling of all the veins. This observation has led him to question the efficacy of treating the long saphenous vein by any means. His method of treatment is by empty-vein technique in which the needle is introduced into the enlarged vein with the patient sitting, after which the leg is elevated with the patient lying down, and 0.5 c.c. of 3% Sotradecol is injected into the empty segment, using finger pressure to localize the solution in the emptied vein. This is similar to the techniques mentioned above.

I have always made it a practice to inject perforator veins whenever they were present.

There are two ways of making these injections. One is to inject the perforators in the standing or sitting position, the latter being preferred. Here the needle finds the opening of the vein where it meets the superficial branch that feeds it. The stream is often reversed, and its rapidity can be gauged by the reflux of blood into the syringe that the operator is holding. If there is not much pressure in the venous stream, the plunger will stay in position and an ordinary varicose vein injection will probably suffice. In these instances, the operator must be careful not to inject a large amount of sclerosing fluid which may travel into the deep veins and cause a deep venous thrombosis. With a greater degree of backflow from the perforator being treated, it may be necessary to increase the volume of the injected solution in order to fill the perforator blood vessel and secure sclerosis. Again, the dosage depends upon clinical experience as there is no standard amount for each case. A further control of the sclerosing efficiency for this injection treatment will be afforded by the position of the patient. Thus, the patient may be kept standing, sitting, or the leg may be elevated for this injection. This will depend upon the judgment of the operator.

With increasing knowledge, based upon experience, it is a good idea for the operator in this field to train himself and give these injections with the patient flat on his back and the limb elevated to an upright position.* In this position palpation will demonstrate the openings of the perforator channels as indentations which become more recognizable with practice. This is the ideal position for perforator vein treatment as it also tends to empty these veins. The dose of medication will vary depending upon the size and location of these communicating veins. When one considers that these branches must be sclerosed inward toward the deep system, it is obvious that a meticulous technique must be practiced. The area of the vein must be isolated by digital pressure which should be about two inches. One-half c.c. of Sotradecol is injected while the finger pressure is maintained for about a minute. After this, the leg is lowered and pressure bandages are applied.

Compression Sclerotherapy

Compression has been the rule since the beginning of varicose vein therapy. The mainstay of the early forms of pressure has been, and still is, the gauze sponge. This is something that has never been available commercially but has to be made by hand utilizing gauze squares of two sizes. For the average varicose vein injection, one utilizes nine inch squares of gauze. These are folded in half and fashioned into compact round gauze sponges. A double layer of gauze is used to shape larger gauze sponges for vein injections, while a single layer is fashioned into a smaller ball of gauze for capillary and small vein injections.

After an ordinary vein injection, one to three or more gauze sponges are placed over the vein that has been treated and held in place by one inch strips of adhesive 9 to 12 inches long. This is repeated for each vein injection at any point on the leg.

Prior to the outset of treatment, each individual who has advanced varicosities must prepare for his treatment by securing an elastic, specially woven stocking or leotard.** These are worn as soon as possible after the initial treatment is concluded. In the meantime it is my practice to bandage the leg firmly with elastic bandages four inches wide up to the knee where they are secured by metal clips. From the knee up I apply another type of four inch bandage*** which is self-adhering in type but does not stick to the skin. This upper bandage may be kept from rolling down by adhesive strapping or by the use of

* As also advocated by Fegan.

** Jobst and others

*** Peg

elastoplast types of elastic bandages which adhere to the skin. Added pressure may be effected by wearing elastic stockings or leotards over the elastic bandages or a double layer of elastic bandages may be used.

There is a large variety of other supports that are used for compression. These vary from country to country. Some of the materials are crepe bandages without rubber, cotton sponges which are placed over the injection sites, preformed molded soft rubber in various shapes to fit over injection sites, foam rubber and sorbo rubber pads. These can be trimmed to shape by the operator to prevent skin abrasion or irritation under the knee and in the upper thigh near the groin. The variety of stockings and waist high elastic garments is bewildering in its numbers. The operator must show ingenuity in arriving at a solution for compressing each case. The patient must be coached to cooperate by keeping support bandaging on as prescribed. In all cases, patients are ordered, unquestionably, to be ambulatory.

The length of compression time depends upon the severity of the varicose condition. Patients with superficial veins and no major reflux need to wear compression bandages for three to four weeks. When incompetence of the saphenous or perforator system has occurred, compression must be maintained for a minimum of six weeks. Bandages may be removed for each treatment day, as outlined below, and often the same bandages can be applied following each day of injection. Any slipping of the bandages must be corrected immediately.

Rapid Treatment

A typical plan of treatment for a three-day concentrated case is as follows:

First Day of Treatment

A complete and careful history is taken. Special inquiry is made regarding previous allergies or attacks of phlebitis.

A special physical examination should include testing for arterial adequacy and incompetent veins in the saphenous and perforator vein systems. The lower abdomen and genitalia should be checked for varicosities.

Small venule enlargements and capillary dilatations should be recorded. Phlebosclerosis or calcification may be present in long-standing varicosities. The usual check should be made of thyroid hyperactivity, acute infections, and advanced constitutional diseases. Diabetes should be brought under control. In general, it is astonishing how very few individuals have had to be excluded from taking varicose vein treatment because of contraindications.

If the history and physical examination are negative, rapid treatment may be commenced immediately. The therapist should make an immediate provocative injection of 1 c.c. 50% glucose solution. Other first solutions are invert sugar 60% or mixtures of salt and sugar, like dextrose 25% with sodium chloride 10%. Any of these three bland solutions may be used as the initial injection. Since these patients are usually kept in the office all day, this test may be read within three hours. Latent or mild phlebitis will be indicated by a painful or spreading reaction in the treated vein. If there is no reaction, rapid treatment may continue immediately.

In cases of doubt regarding phlebitis, the therapist may perform an erythrocyte sedimentation test. There will invariably be a definite increase in the sedimentation rate when a phlebitic infection is present (20).

That same day, a few hours later at the second session, a few minims of sodium morrhuate are injected. This is a test for allergy to fatty acid solutions in general. This test is examined in one of two ways, depending upon the arrangement of the office schedule. The operator may wait an hour or three hours, depending upon his plans for that case. If he decides to check the injection in one hour, he will examine the patient at the time for signs of allergy. This may be indicated by localized itching or perhaps a greater reaction with whealing. Occasionally, a nervous patient may have bizarre symptoms which are unrelated to the actual injection. This may be in the form of nausea, giddiness, flushing, or perhaps a feeling of faintness. The operator will quickly learn to distinguish between these nervous symptoms and true allergy. To avoid some of the false responses, I always advise my patients to eat some solid food prior to treatment, and I expressly state that it consist of eggs, meat, sandwichs, and not just toast and coffee. This will eliminate many threatened attacks of syncope or nausea.

If there is no allergy, the operator can inject 0.5 c.c. of sodium morrhuate in the third session. He may also introduce another sclerosing agent, like 0.5 to 1 c.c. Sotradecol 3%, at this time.

If he elects to wait three hours before reading the test for allergy, he will then give the above two injections three hours later.

We have now given the patient the initial provocative injection, followed by a second test injection for allergy, succeeded by a third session in which the patient receives an increased dosage of sodium morrhuate plus a second sclerosing agent, in this case Sotradecol 3%.

Experienced operators, especially with a large volume of patients, may only treat the patient in two sessions on the first treatment day. There must be a pause of approximately three hours between the provocative injection and the test for allergy. However, if the history indicates and the operator feels that there is little possibility of allergic manifestation, he can make the second treatment 0.5 to 1 c.c. of sodium morrhuate, instead of just injecting a few minims, and will thereby get the case started a little faster. There is usually no time on the first treatment day to study the patient's vein reaction. However, if there is time, another treatment session may be arranged two or three hours later in order to appraise the effect of the second sclerosing session. It is often not necessary to carry the treatment beyond this point on the first day. However, if the case is a large one, a third injection session may be advisable.

The patient is given instructions about hygiene following this treatment and urged to walk and move around in order to keep the blood in circulation. The application of an ice bag in the area of treatment will control any tenderness he may develop.

It is usually not necessary on the first day of treatment to use anything but gauze ball sponges and strips of adhesive over the veins. However, one may begin at this point to employ some mild form of compression bandage to keep the superficial venous tree flattened.

Second Day of Treatment

By now the patient has had two or three testing sessions which are also beginning treatments, and it is now possible to start full-dosage therapy. The same general rules for therapy in the slower conservative technique still apply here but in a more rapid fashion. Thus one can give full-sized treatments to the leg veins on the first office session that day, and continue with the saphenous veins on the second visit that day. Whenever feasible, empty-vein techniques should be employed to reduce the incidence of bulky, painful thromboses which slow up healing and cause needless suffering.

There can be two or three sessions on this second day of treatment, and the solutions used will depend upon the responses to the previous injections.

The reactions to the second day of treatment may be extremely gratifying and reduce the rest of the case to simple proportions. Before the patient is sent home, provision is made for adequate compression of the treated areas as well as untreated veins which may feed these areas to cause recanalization.

It is my practice to thoroughly compress enlarged saphenous systems, leg veins, and perforators before sending the patient home the second day. I employ gauze sponges and adhesive strips, foam rubber sheets and pads, four-inch elastic bandages, elastic adhesive bandages, and four-inch bandages – the latter being a modified elastic bandage which adheres to itself but not the skin of the patient.

If the patient has an advanced case with large incompetent veins, a well-fitting, gradient pressure elastic support will have been prescribed. These supports in full length form or leotard arrangement should be ordered in advance so they can be used early in the treatment. Sometimes, embolism stockings or conventional elastic stockings are temporarily used if gradient stockings are not immediately available to compress the incompetent varicosities of the limb.

Whatever form of pressure is used, it must be adequate and worn constantly until the next treatment session, which is usually two days later. When the patient leaves, he is given a prescription for 100 mg. of Butazolidin* in the event he has exaggerated inflammatory responses. Only a few patients fill these prescriptions, as the majority are not uncomfortable with this treatment plan. The patients are instructed not to rest in bed during the daytime, but to carry on normal activity as ambulation definitely favors healing. Very few patients fail to carry out these instructions as they are given them in pamphlet form for better compliance. Patients are also cautioned against excessive muscular activity such as tennis, golf, horseback riding, jogging, gymnastics, bicycle riding, and skating. Whirlpool baths and massages are absolutely forbidden.

Third Day of Treatment

The bandages are now removed and the patient's reactions are carefully checked. Remaining varicosities are marked by ball-point pen for empty-vein techniques wherever needed. Smaller veins are treated in the usual stand-up fashion or sitting techniques. Some cosmetic work can be done at this time including dilated venules. Capillaries have to be reserved for a subsequent treatment (Chapter 13).

During the three sessions remaining on the third day, it should be possible to complete the average case. This may mean as many as six injections at each session, if needed. In order to give this many treatments, it will be necessary to have available a variety of sclerosing agents, as using the same solution may exceed the recommended dosage for one day. Thus, for example, 10 to 15 injections may be given on this third day divided among three sclerosing agents; sodium morrhuate, Sotradecol, and 50% glucose.

For the occasional case where large thrombi are formed with painful perivenous induration, while the condition will be absorbed normally, the discomfort may be quickly relieved by removing some of the clot. Some practitioners do this by making an incision over the vein and shelling out the actual clot. The author prefers to use a large bore 13 gauge needle with which he can aspirate some of the liquid in the clot and expel the balance by squeezing it through the needle opening between two gauze sponges.

The patient is cautioned again against excessive exercise, and conversely, against excessive rest in the daytime. Care must be observed that total compression of all the treated veins is accomplished by the bandaging that is applied. Many patients will not submit to continuous total bandaging for six weeks to several months. A practical compromise must be found in the form of

*Dolobid Tablets (Diflunisal, M.S.D.) 250 mgms, may be substituted.

elastic bandaging, stockings, or leotards to maintain compression while the sclerosed vein segments are becoming fibrotic or disintegrate. This may require some ingenuity on the part of the operator.

There are a group of patients who are advised to wear elastic stockings for a period of six months to a year or more. These are patients with enlarged legs due to complicating advanced lymphedema or incompetent deep venous systems.

Venules and Capillaries

Consideration must be given even in these rapid cases to the treatment of capillaries and venules. It is very seldom that capillary enlargements can be treated simultaneously with the varicosities. Generally a special arrangement must be made to treat these finest blood vessels later, after healing of the main veins. Venules, however, can often be treated immediately, especially if they are bulging and protrude above the skin surface. Some of the flat, fine venules may have to be postponed to be done along with the capillaries at a later date. Blotches may be treated with the capillaries (see Chapter 14, Cosmetic Aspects).

Chapter 6

▪ COMPLICATIONS ACCOMPANYING VARICOSE VEINS

The complications of varicose veins that will be described here are varicose eczema, skin allergies, pigmentation, sloughing, and embolism. The conditions of varicose ulcer and unilateral enlargement are considered separately under their own headings in Chapters 8 and 12. These skin complications of varicose veins may be present prior to injection treatment or may occur after treatment.

Eczema

Sutton* describes eczema as an acute or chronic inflammatory disease characterized by erythema, papules, vesicles, pustules, scales, and scabs. These lesions are found alone or combined with skin thickening. This thickening and infiltration is accompanied by itching and burning in many cases. Sutton goes on to say, "It is not possible to formulate a satisfactory definition of this disorder or to state precisely what the term does include or does not include." If the reader would like a convenient two-word definition that would apply to every case, it would be a "dermatologic scrap-heap."

Dorland** describes eczema as an inflammatory skin disease with vesiculation, infiltration, watery discharge, and the development of scales and crusts. McPheeters (21) states that the continued congestion of the skin in varicose veins causes a very intense dermatitis that later may become the most extensive, moist, and oozing type of lesion. This is frequently associated with ringworm of the foot, the combination being sometimes termed eczematoid ringworm. The confusing array of names for these skin conditions is rendered more distracting by the fact that various authors referring to the same conditions may use different terms.

---

* Sutton – Handbook of Diseases of the Skin. 1949.

** Medical Dictionary

It is important to keep in mind that we are dealing with common skin conditions occurring on a background of chronic venous stasis making the usual pattern of familiar skin diseases take on a different aspect because of the stagnant circulation. In fact, a whole new text book of skin diseases could, and perhaps should, be written describing the skin picture as a result of the disturbed circulation in varicose veins.

An ordinary dermatitis may look entirely different on such a leg, and it takes considerable experience for the observer to recognize the condition. While an acute eczema occurring on a normal leg may be fiery red with copious weeping; in the presence of indolent venous flow, it might assume a much paler color with less moisture.

The pathology occurs in the upper skin layers and consists of spongiosis, acanthosis, parakerotosis, and in the cutis propria, hyperemia, edema, and moderate cell infiltration. The eruptions which take place may be acute or recurrent. They show a tendency to arrange themselves in spots, plaques, or large patches with irregular contours.

Subjectively, eczema or dermatitis is accompanied by itching and burning. Often itching is the first symptom that brings the patient to the doctor's office for relief. He has noted that applying ointments has not effected a cure. It will be necessary for the physician to relieve the venous stagnation in order to correct the skin condition. The whole group of skin diseases accompanying varicose veins must thus be treated for the venous stasis along with the standard skin therapy to restore normalcy.

In neglected cases, after long periods of time, these skin lesions are in a stubborn phase of inactivity from which they are roused with some difficulty. This is especially the case where regeneration of new skin is needed for healing.

Treatment of Dermatitis and Eczema

Injection treatment of the varicose background is the first step in the healing process. Minor or early lesions usually respond promptly to the restoration of the normal venous flow. Itching promptly ceases.

Where the varicose eczema has been of long standing, it often shows fibrous induration around the edges and underneath the lesion. This wall which has developed seals the lesion and prevents it from spreading further, but also chokes off the epithelial tissues' microscopic vascular supply. Chronic cases may have avascular walls and bases precluding normal nourishment to the epithelial and, sometimes, subcutaneous tissues involved. I have noticed the similarity between these indurated walls and the induration around ulcers occurring in lymphedema, which has inspired the injection treatment described below.

It is only suitable where fibrous induration exists and is not recommended for superficial eczema in the acute vesicular stage, as the tissues are too delicate to tolerate injections.

First, the varicosities are treated in the usual fashion. When the veins are finished, the eczematous skin is started. After preliminary skin anesthesia with Procaine or Xylocaine, a 20 gauge 1½ inch needle containing isotonic mixtures of Ringer's solution or normal saline is injected as in lymph ulcer (Chapter 12). The needle is started in healthy tissue and carried subcutaneously into and through the ring of induration surrounding the skin condition. The needles are directed into the deeper areas of the skin and subcutaneous tissues if needed. The entire wall of induration must be traversed, ending in healthy tissue.

The entire circle of induration, if present, should be injected in this fashion, fanning out from the point of entry of the needle in order to minimize the number of injections beginning in the healthy skin.

The walls of indurated or fibrotic tissue are thus perforated and infiltrated with isotonic solution, which acts as channels for capillary and lymph flow in the area. Furthermore, it has been demonstrated that this treatment stimulates the growth of new capillary and lymph blood vessels. (45) These injection treatments may be given weekly until healing takes place.

The above injections are followed by gauze bandaging with a soothing ointment dressing such as Lassar's Plain Paste, or other suitable ointment. With large weeping lesions of the skin it may be necessary to follow the treatment with unna paste bandages until healing occurs.

The results have been gratifying and conclusive. Areas of stubborn eczema or dermatitis that have been associated with varicose veins for many years have been treated successfully. Lesions where great thickening and, perhaps, pigmentation has occurred after years of scratching, also react positively to this therapy. While some individuals do not obtain complete removal of the unsightly lesions, even these cases show marked improvement. The majority respond by complete healing and only rarely is skin grafting needed to complete the cure.

The first effects noted are the loss of the scaly epidermis and the weeping character of the skin. The surface of the area becomes smoother and drier. Itching is relieved but does not always subside at the outset. Sometimes the injections have to be supplemented by antipruritic ointment as dressing where needed. The types of eczema that respond the best are those patchy types which have definite induration and thickening in the deeper epithelial tissues. It is here that the injections best perform their function of providing a healthy base for the growth of a new capillary and lymph circulation.

Where the skin practically rests on the periosteum as over the malleoli in the ankle region, a difficult problem ensues. One cannot pierce this skin or flood under it by the same technique. A subcutaneous base is a minimal prerequisite for this injection treatment. Sometimes by using tiny 27 or 30 gauge needles one can actually perform micro-injections and try to infiltrate the very scanty subcutaneous layer of the eczema area. Prompt healing will take place if one has sufficient tissue to work on.

Skin Allergies

Allergic reactions are the dangerous episodes of sclerotherapy in varicose veins. Every effort should be made to avoid this complication. Prevention is the best treatment, and the first step is the case history. This must emphasize the following points:

1) A description of prior injections, their purpose, medications used, and special emphasis on previous allergic reactions;

2) A previous background of hayfever, bronchial asthma, eczema, angioneurotic edema, hives, migraine, or gastrointestinal allergic upsets;

3) A family history of allergy;

4) A careful inquiry into drug sensitivities aside from allergy and how they were manifested.

This kind of careful history will, in the great majority of patients, detect allergy-prone individuals who can be treated with extra caution.

Careful questioning may bring out the possible development of cross allergies. Thus, a fish sensitivity, as an example, may produce an allergic response during the patient's treatment following the injection of sodium morrhuate which is a cod liver oil extract.

The usual skin tests performed by an allergist cannot be relied upon in the case of intravenous therapy. The reactions obtained by patch, oral, or conjunctival methods have been tried by me and do not always give a clue as to what might develop following intravenous injection.

The best test is the clinical test, and I strongly recommend that extreme caution be observed in beginning the usual case, especially in individuals who are suspect. It is dangerous to start any case of varicose veins with a full dose of any sclerosing solution that may have traces of protein in its composition. In fact, there have been instances where synthetic chemicals that apparently have no protein whatsoever in their make-up have produced allergic responses.

It must be kept in mind that rarely can one get a full-blown allergic reaction following the injection of the most innocent of sclerosing solutions. Furthermore, we are all familiar with those individuals who develop giant urticaria without any discernible cause at all. The whole subject of allergies following injection treatment needs continued study; nevertheless, it remains clear that the more care the operator observes, the less frequently will allergy occur. In my experience generalized, constitutional reactions have become so rare in my later years as to be practically non-existent. This is the result, not only of effectively choosing safe solutions, but also reflects the result of calming and reassuring even the most apprehensive of individuals.

As discussed in Chapters 4 and 5, the first three injections should be very guarded. This holds true whether the earlier standard technique is used or the newer rapid injection method. I never use anything but sugar or salt solutions as the first injection. This helps to rule out latent or quiescent phlebitis. The second injection is carefully chosen with allergy in mind. If the patient gives a history of possible or actual sensitivity or allergy to a specific chemical or group of chemicals, the physican should try to avoid these substances completely and treat the patient with another type of sclerosing agent. If a fatty acid solution like sodium morrhuate has caused previous allergic responses, it is expedient to avoid the whole family of fatty acid solutions. There can never be too may sclerosing agents at hand. In a large practice, there will always be some individuals who require special medication, and the operator with a large armamentarium of sclerosing agents can always find at least one that is safe for that particular case.

Sensitization may have taken place in patients who have never had preceding varicose vein therapy. It is here that an allergic response may occur with the very first injection. At other times, sensitization may develop during the course of treatment. This is especially likely to happen if several injections of a substance that the patient is allergic to are followed by a pause of weeks or months. After such a hiatus, if the same solution is used again, reactions may occur. During the interval, the body has an opportunity to develop antibodies or reagins which cause the release of histamine and the ensuing allergic symptoms. It is well to emphasize, at this point, the interesting fact that my rapid method of treatment described in Chapter 5 has practically eliminated allergic reactions because the body fluids don't have sufficient time to elaborate antibodies.

An alert operator will be on guard for early symptoms of impending allergy. A premonitory warning which usually precedes attacks would be areas of localized itching or skin rashes. Even if these are coincidental or questionable, it is better to change solutions than risk a major allergy. Again, the doctor with a variety of sclerosing agents at hand is in a favorable position to make these necessary changes.

The doctor who practices the treatment of varicose veins on a large scale will be impressed by the number of individuals who become temporarily ill following initial injections. Sometimes it is difficult to differentiate between allergic responses, neurotic reactions, and frank hysteria. These responses are always intensified if the patient reports for treatment without having some food in his stomach. I, therefore, make it a practice to insist that everyone undergoing this therapy must eat within an hour prior to treatment. I emphasize that this food should be solid and substantial and not just a cup of coffee or a slice of toast. A sign with this warning should be displayed conspicuously near the area of treatment so that every patient is suitably informed.

The presence of digestive products in the blood stream act as a buffer minimizing the impact of the injected medication. Without previous eating, symptoms such as nausea, giddiness, and mild circulatory collapse often occur in patients who have not had sufficient breakfast. This is so well marked that the correlation is clear.

It must be added that hypertensives sometimes react even in the absence of true allergy. They are the ones who may develop a generalized flush even with sugar solutions. This is a vasomotor disturbance and not real allergy.

The operator, in these cases, should check the patient, and if the conjuctiva are not congested, reassure the patient that it is only a minor upset. Almost always, patients who feel faint or develop a flush are quickly relieved by lying down on the examining table and being exposed to fresh air. If these measures afford quick relief, it is a further confirmation of the fact that the reaction is not truly allergic.

Another, sometimes difficult, differentiation must be made between chemical sensitivity and true allergy. For instance, quinine and urethane may be responsible for confusing symptoms in susceptible patients. In some individuals, the injection of 1 or 2 c.c.'s of this solution may cause transitory flushing, dizziness, and a sensation of warmth in the throat. Some patients may taste the medication. This series of symptoms are due to mild sensitivity to quinine. More severe symptoms following quinine administration include nausea, persistent vertigo, and intestinal or uterine spasm. Sometimes females may have vaginal bleeding or prolongation of a menstrual period. Cinchonism, in this more serious form, is a signal to change the medication.

On the other hand, major crises can also occur with Quinine especially in hypertensives who may develop shock, or circulatory and respiratory collapse. There may be no preceding warning symptoms. No doctor, doing this therapy, should ever be without a fresh supply of Adrenalin and other emergency drugs, including steroids, for injection as these may be life saving.

The most common allergic response that annoys patients following treatment is the development of skin rash. It becomes necessary to distinguish between the rash resulting from the adhesive strapping and allergic rashes. The conformity of the rash to the line of the adhesive plaster should serve to distinguish between the two. It is only rarely that an adhesive rash may spread over the body, but it can occur. The diagnostic difficulty is then increased, but an experienced operator will recognize the migration of the rash as evidence of contact dermatitis which responds to steroid therapy.

Generalized allergic responses to injection treatment may occur within minutes or up to several hours. One will encounter stoic individuals who will not report warning signals like itching, headaches, nausea, or other discomforts and who will leave the office only to develop an attack while en route to some other destination. This is extremely rare, but the doctor and his staff must always be alert to premonitory symptoms as early signs of possible allergies. I frequently tell my assistants not to let patients who are suspect out of the office until enough time has elapsed to make certain there is no allergic aftermath. An alert staff is of the utmost importance in this respect because patients may disclose symptoms to an office aide that he would not impart to the doctor.

Treatment of Allergic Reactions

If the symptoms are not of a major nature, it is often possible to avert serious allergic responses by the immediate injection of 1 to 5 c.c. of Benadryl solution, intramuscularly. This is not as rapidly acting as other agents, but it will control mild reactions successfully. Patients should be warned that this antihistamine injection may cause drowsiness so that driving a car should be avoided for the next few hours.

The question of whether to lie the patient down or sit him up is answered by the judgment of the operator. In general, it is best to lie the patient down, give him air from an open window or air conditioner, make the proper injection, and most important of all, assume an attitude of confidence or even leave the room temporarily to show the patient that the situation is not serious. I never permit a relative or close friend of the patient to enter the room at this point and build up nervous tension.

If Benadryl does not prevent an attack, or if alarming symptoms develop quickly, one must immediately inject Adrenalin 1:1000. This is done subcutaneously, and the initial dose should be 2 to 3 minims. The patient is given a small sponge and instructed to gently massage the area of injection. This is done so that the vasoconstriction that occurs, which prevents absorption of the

Adrenalin, will be relieved, thereby permitting continued absorption. It is not good therapy, in most cases, to inject 1 c.c. immediately.

After waiting a few minutes, and with proper reassurance and fresh air – which might also include having the assistant sponge the face with cold water – if the symptoms do not abate, a second injection must be made. This time 0.25 to 0.5 c.c. may be administered, again with reassurances. In all, 1 c.c. total dosage of Adrenalin may be used.

Other drugs that may be needed include Decadron or other steroids, Coramine, Ephedrine, Cardilate, Chlortrimeton injectable, or other life-saving drugs that should be available in the doctor's office. One may not see a desperate case in a lifetime of practice, but if oxygen is not available, or even if it is present, the doctor should always be in a position to call the emergency services that are available in his community. These rescue squads may come from fire departments, police departments, and, of course, the nearest hospital. In the meantime, whatever measures may be needed like mouth-to-mouth resuscitation, or artificial respiration, should be used until help arrives. If conditions warrant it, rapid transfer to the emergency room of a nearby hospital may be needed. This has never been necessary in my experience.

The therapist in this field must have at hand safe solutions that he can use for allergic individuals. These solutions, while they are bland and less irritating, may successfully complete a case if necessary. They include dextrose, invert sugar, sodium chloride, and mixtures of dextrose and sodium chloride. Sometimes, the operator may have to employ concentrated sodium salicylate, Scleremo, Variglobin, or Aethoxysklerol. Occasionally, a solution like Quinine which causes allergy in one individual may work out perfectly for another patient. The thing to remember is that there is always a sclerosing solution available for every allergic individual.

By far, the majority of people undergoing treatment tolerate sclerosing solutions without reactions. Only a relatively small allergic group requires these special techniques and solutions. In spite of the fact that an average generalist doing this work may never encounter a case with significant allergy, it is essential that all the precautions outlined above be observed.

Pigmentation

This is an annoying complication which cannot be totally eliminated. With clinical experience the doctor may be able to minimize, subdue, or eliminate this reaction in most cases. However, there is a hard core of individuals with a pronounced tendency to deposit melanin in the deep layers of the skin who must be treated guardedly.

This vulnerable group of people who are usually pronounced brunettes possess a lot of pigmentation in their skin which may be provoked into laying down additional pigment granules in the event of skin irritation. This irritation may be in the form of actinic rays or chemical irritation of sclerotherapy. It is essentially a tanning action, but sometimes may stop short to form freckles as a minor pigmentary response.

I have noticed in my work on skin capillaries that there is a most curious and heretofore unpublished association between freckling and telangiectasia. It seems as if some form of irritation, perhaps excessive exposure to sunshine, has stimulated not only the skin but also the capillaries underneath it to form a progressive and closely linked skin blemish. In confirmation of this observation, I have also noted that treatment of the dilated capillaries (Chapter 13) in these patients concomitantly removes the freckles in that area. I can find no explanation for this linkage.

The most annoying form of pigmentation is found in those individuals who have dark brunette or black hair and dark-toned skin. These patients may develop, after injection-treatment of varicose veins, an objectionable dark brownish to black skin discoloration, usually confined to the location and size of the blood vessel treated. Patients who develop pronounced inflammatory reactions to sclerotherapy are particularly prone to this complication. The pigmentation may occur rapidly, within a few weeks, or take a longer period to develop. It is often possible to reduce or eliminate this unfavorable reaction by using the sclerosing solution in a more dilute form for subsequent injections.

Operators usually find that the skin of susceptible patients will tolerate a dilution up to a certain point, after which tanning or pigmentation occurs. An alert physician will stay within the skin tolerance of the patient. Early warning signals should occur in most cases, and the operator who is aware of this will modify the sclerosing solution early in the case. Practitioners in this area of medicine quickly learn that dark brunettes are prone to pigmentation and, therefore, sclerotherapy for these individuals should be started at the lower limit of tolerance. Sometimes, it may not be possible to find a solution that is effective without pigmenting the patient. In these cases the solution should be changed to a different type which is less prone to cause pigmentary results (see Chapter 13).

Pigmentation, following injection treatment, has a tendency to fade with time and disappear spontaneously. There has been some work recently on the use of Heparin ointment rubbed into the skin prior to injection to control pigmentation, but it has not produced predictable results up to the present. The employment of bleaching creams to hasten the depigmentation is, however,

* Private communication from Ken P. Biegeleisen M.D. N.Y.C. 1983.

well established and may be prescribed by the attending physician. The most efficient of these preparations is Soloquin.* If bleaching creams are not used, most pigment spots or streaks will fade naturally within a period of one to four years.

Sloughing

A formidable complication of injection treatment for varicose veins is the development of skin sloughs. This most annoying outcome needs to be understood thoroughly by the doctor attempting this therapy. Some solutions are especially prone to cause skin necrosis. Unfortunately, it is a complication that may occur in good hands under apparently ideal conditions.

The chemical that is injected produces its effects by several types of tissue irritation, as described in Chapter 3. While the aim of the treament is to limit the irritation to the intima of the blood vessel that is being treated, this is sometimes impossible to achieve. In locations like the skin around the ankle and the dorsum of the foot, or over the bony areas of the leg, there is insufficient sub-epithelial tissues to cushion the effect of the injection. The skin almost rests upon the periostium of the bone in these areas, and the inflammatory response to the injected solution may involve the skin which lies in close opposition to the vein. Furthermore, at the bottom of the leg the venous pressure is at its highest and the venous circulation is at its slowest which makes this area more vulnerable due to increased tissue fragility. I often advise using the mildest sclerosing solutions in these weak areas.

Another way of inadvertently getting a slough, in spite of a good injection, is for the solution to leak back along the needle tract, thereby irritating the skin (Fig. 11). This is more likely to occur if the operator has punctured the vein in several places while attempting to make the injection. Of course, at all costs, the operator must never make a perivascular injection while treating varicose veins. If he finds this has occurred, he must rapidly take the following steps to avert necrosis.

1) Immediately aspirate as much solution as possible, even though it is blood tinged. This will remove some of the extravasated sclerosing solution from the area immediately.

2) Quickly flood the area with 2 to 5 c.c. of Procaine or Xylocaine solution. Distribute the anesthetic solution over a wide area encompassing the

---

*Elder Pharmaceutical Co., Bryan, Ohio.

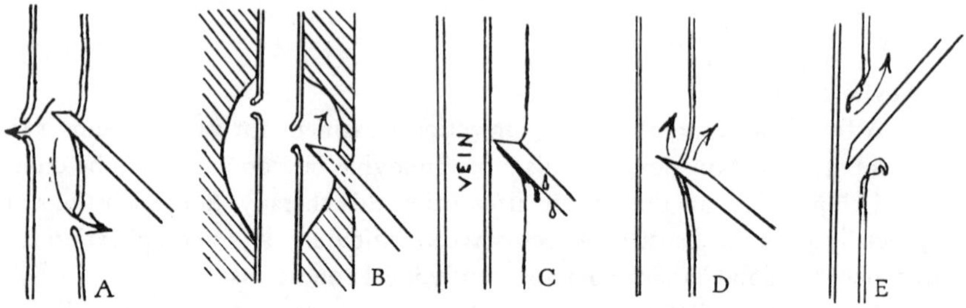

Figure 11. Shows the possibility of perivascular irritation and slough formation even though blood is aspirated by the syringe. A. Needle in vein, solution leaks out through previous holes. B. Needle in hematoma. C. Solution on needle itself irritating needle track. D. Bevel of needle partly in and partly out of vein. E. Solution escaping from torn vein.

injection site. This will cause vasodilation, relax spasm, and promote the rapid dispersal of the irritating fluid. It usually suffices to neutralize the irritation of the offending sclerosing solution. Another good measure to employ is to also flood the area with normal saline solution in amounts up to 20 c.c., depending upon the amount and placement of the sclerosing treatment. Massage and pinching of the tissues manually is also of some assistance.

These measures are aimed at preventing slough formation. However, if necrosis does occur, if may result in a small skin blister or more seriously a larger necrotic area. It is of the utmost importance, when this complication occurs, to have your patient follow these instructions.

A simple blister is usually emptied after pricking it open with a sterile needle. It is then dressed with a sterile dry bandage or bandaid. Sometimes the skin is painted with tincture of merthiolate.

For the more serious larger slough, I insist upon total asepsis and antiseptic dressings held in place by elastic bandages. Occasionally, the edges of the necrotic area may be coapted with flamed adhesive, or perhaps an actual suture to bring the edges together. These sloughs are notoriously slow to heal and will tax the patience of both doctor and patient. However, ordinary antiseptic measures and occasionally a soothing ointment containing an antibiotic will assist the healing. Sloughs invariably yield to these simple measures, during which the patient must be encouraged to follow instructions. It is especially important to avoid salt water bathing during these episodes.

Pulmonary Embolism

This is a life-threatening complication of sclerotherapy for varicose veins, whose frequency has been exaggerated. It is no longer dreaded because it is becoming increasingly rare due to improved treatment. In my experience of 50 years, I have encountered it six times. There were no fatalities.

The occurrence of pulmonary embolus is still unpredictable. In previous years it sometimes occurred in cases of phlebitis that developed large thromboses following injections in distended veins. On the other hand, I have observed it in cases that did not have phlebitis or large saphenous veins and who were apparently healing smoothly without incident.

Theoretically its origin may arise from an extension of the sclerosing reaction into the deep tibial or femoral veins. I have traced other attacks to unusual muscular exertion or, conversely, to too little physical activity.

Its diagnosis, while still difficult, has been improved by advances in knowledge of the enzymes in blood serum, and also by lung scanning and x-ray tomography. While the treatment of embolism is not within the scope of this manual of ambulatory sclerotherapy, it should be noted that this condition may yield to the technique of dissolving blood clots by the intravenous infusion of streptokinase and thrombokinase. The basis of hospital treatment still rests on anticoagulant therapy with surgery reserved for cases that exhibit recurring embolic attacks.

Prevention of Pulmonary Embolism

The first step in prevention is the avoidance of large, bulky reactions to sclerotherapy. This requires a knowledge of proper sclerosing procedures and solutions, and the utilization of empty-vein techniques for appropriate large veins.

Compression of treated veins is the next step in prophylaxis of embolism. While compression, in some form, has been an essential part of the therapy for varicose veins since its infancy, recent emphasis on a six week continuous pressure bandaging technique further reduces the probability of this complication developing (see Chapter 5).

Proper exercise is the third step in treatment. This can be provided in many ways with walking and swimming leading the list. Strenuous muscular activity should be restricted for one month after injection treatment. Activities like tennis, handball, jogging, and even golf are curtailed for this period. Horseback riding especially is not permitted for six weeks until the veins have completely healed.

The patient is instructed in the use of elastic stockings and the different varieties of self-adhering bandages as well as elastic adhesive (see Chapter 5).

The prevention of embolus, therefore, lies with the correct application of sclerosing techniques, followed by appropriate methods of securing compression or effacement of the superficial venous tree until the treated veins have healed and have been absorbed by the body.

Chapter 7

▪ PHLEBITIS IN VARICOSE VEINS

Phlebitis in varicose veins is an inflammation of the vein wall occurring in the presence of a stagnant or reverse circulation. On the other hand, phlebitis found in a normal superficial vein develops in spite of a normal blood flow travelling in the right direction, toward the heart. This makes for two diverse types of origin and there are, therefore, two methods of treatment.

Etiology

The etiology of varicose phlebitis has not been established, although the probable causes have been discussed by many observers, and the literature is replete with their theories. Hume (22) writes of the deficiency in our understanding about pathophysiology in thrombophlebitis, which is true about all of the thrombotic conditions. This deficiency contributes to inaccurate diagnosis. He further suggests that in discussing etiology a triad of factors is usually mentioned. These are stasis or turbulence, a *vascular* factor, and some blood factor. Blood tests have resulted in disagreement as to whether a blood factor has been measured. His tests could not demonstrate any difference between superficial thrombophlebitis and the deep variety.

Maciej Szczepanski (23) investigated forty-five patients with superficial thrombophlebitis, some of whom received sclerosing injections while others had spontaneous inflammation. After a study of the blood findings, he concluded that the laboratory determinations of the clotting time, fibrinogen level, heparin tolerance, and clot lysis time did not disclose any diagnostically significant findings in superficial thrombophlebitis in any case.

In recent years it has become evident that during the administration of oral contraceptives, a higher incidence of superficial thrombophlebitis was found in women with varicose veins.

There is universal agreement that whatever factors are involved in the production of superficial thrombophlebitis, the presence of the stagnant blood stream makes varicose veins especially prone to clotting or inflammation.

On the other hand, there are conditions in which apparantly normal superficial veins become inflamed for no discernible cause. It is even more mystifying when phlebitis occurs in the deep system of veins in the lower extremity.

We have looked for the answer to the problem of phlebitis by searching for and trying to identify bacteria or viruses, and have not been able to find any consistant etiologic infecting organism to explain the onset of these inflammations. DeTakats (24) cultured bacteria from isolated vein segments that he excised in a general group of varicose vein cases. He reported a slow growing bacterial growth of low virulence in five to ten days in half of his cases. This corresponds clinically with the *flare-ups* I have observed following injection treatment in these cases. They followed an incubation period resembling that in deTakat's cultures. This has never been confirmed by any other investigators. Practically all observers agree that the veins and clots in superficial phlebitis do not harbor bacteria. More work is needed in this area.

Half of all varicose vein patients harbor infection in the dilated venous system, and treatment must take into account this factor. The frequency and progress of these phlebitides are not appreciated, but they are of enormous significance. The steady progression of inevitable infection in the varicosed extremity can be expressed by a pattern which can be formulated as follows:

Varicose Veins   Latent Phlebitis   Acute Varico-phlebitis

Accompanying Lymphangitis   Lymphedema (Lymph Leg)

This series of infections, once begun, if unchecked becomes irreversible and goes on to its end stage of lymph leg in time. The time span may be five to twenty years, but is inevitable unless checked by the resistance of the patient or appropriate treatment (see Chapter 12).

Types of Phlebitis in Varicose Veins

The recognizable varieties of phlebitis accompanying varicose veins are the hyperacute or fulminating, acute, latent, and chronic.

The rare hyperacute case resembles the condition occurring in a normal superficial vein that becomes inflamed from trauma or sepsis. This type is dangerous to treat until the inflammation subsides. An injudicious injection in such a hyperacute case may spread rapidly to cause serious effects. These cases are rare and I have not observed any for years. With antibiotics, they do not present a problem, and it is possible that they are caused by secondary bacterial infection. More commonly one sees the typical acute type.

Acute Phlebitis

The typical acute phlebitic attack may begin with the sudden appearance of a hot, painful lump in the lower extremity. If varicosities have previously existed, the patient may notice that one of them has become hard and tender. The clot may be elongated to resemble a small pencil. These painful lumps may appear anywhere on the lower extremity. If it involves the great saphenous vein, the thrombosis may extend the entire length of the thigh and cause only moderate pain and disability – an important point in differentiating from other types of phlebitis.

As an interesting corollary, one must take note of the prevailing fashion to use the great saphenous vein for bypass grafting surgery in coronary artery disease as well as femoro-popliteal disease. *Caution should be observed to avoid grafting a varicosed blood vessel which is so prone to latent infection.*

Latent Phlebitis

Latent phlebitis commonly affects a considerable proportion of varicose veins. Its detection is usually impossible by ordinary examination. Untrained operators may find, in the course of sclerotherapy for varicose veins, that there will occasionally be a marked reaction to an average dose of sclerosing fluid early in the case. Unless they are aware of the possible existence of this type of slumbering infection, they will not understand the nature of the reaction.

Dormant infection in varicose veins deserves more emphasis. Its presence is undeniable to anyone with experience in the vascular field. A specific test for its recognition is described below.

Chronic Phlebitis

Chronic phlebitis is not a clearcut entity in varicose veins. It represents an end stage in cases that have been present for years, and can be identified by the thickened, often calcified, vein walls that are slightly tender to pressure. These thickened veins are also found in areas of lymphedema, and are usually discovered accidentally while injecting lymph areas. Here, the tissues are matted together by an indolent infection in the subcutaneous tissue which traps the superficial veins that they surround.

Diagnosis

While it is not necessary to present a complete classification of all the other types of phlebitis found in the lower extremities, the important ones can be listed at this point. They include migrating phlebitis; phlebitis in specific diseases like syphillis, tuberculosis, and Buerger's disease; phlebitis accompanying malignancy; and phlebitis in miscellaneous diseases like typhoid and influenza.

Most of these do not constitute a problem in differential diagnosis. However, there are three which may cause confusion, and they will be described.

Migrating Phlebitis

This is an indeterminate chronic disease that often recurs but the attacks are usually transient and self-limited. It may appear anywhere on or in the body. The veins that are involved on the surface may appear on the lower extremities and are usually small and insignificant. They are palpable as small lumps affecting the normal veins and not the varicosed vessels. This is the distinguishing point of difference. They should be left alone and not injected because they will disappear within a matter of weeks. They may be an early, or only presenting, sign of an occult visceral malignancy.

Thromboangiitis Obliterans (Buerger's Disease)

This affliction has become more rare in recent years coincidental with the decline in cigarette consumption. It may be recognized by an accompanying migratory form of phlebitis and is often seen in the lower leg and foot. The disease is recognized by measurable arterial impairment, and the special inflammatory lesions which envelope vein, artery, and nerve in a characteristic fashion. Its extreme rarity in women and the development of tissue necrosis and cyanosis of the foot and toes serve for easy identification. There is usually no diagnostic problem.

Phlebitis Accompanying Malignancy

The phlebitis that accompanies malignancy often has no special identifying signs. However, the sudden appearance of venous thrombosis, in normal large or small veins, without any antecedent history should lead the observer to investigate the possibility of new growth. I have never seen this kind of venous thrombosis mistaken for varico-phlebitis, as the presence of other varicose veins on the lower limbs should establish the diagnosis.

Diagnosis of Varico-phlebitis

The obvious type of varicose phlebitis occurs in the case that has the usual picture of varicosities connected with the saphenous vein system. Here, a visible varicosity becomes tender, reddened, and inflamed. This draws the patient's attention to the area. Palpation discloses a hard lump over the vein involved. The patient usually makes the diagnosis himself without medical assistance. With greater involvement, the picture is similarly clear.

Examination of the larger trunks in the thigh involving the greater saphenous medially, and the lesser on the lateral side, will reveal thrombotic attacks of varying size. In major attacks the large trunk may be thrombosed for its entire length with varying degrees of inflammation. In extensive episodes, the degree of pain and tenderness, with accompanying redness and heat, makes the condition an alarming one. On the other hand, only a small segment of this large vein may be minimally inflamed so that the resulting thrombosis is not noticeable.

The problem cases are those where a mild thrombophlebitic process occurs in one small varicose vein. Here, the pain and tenderness is of a mild nature and is often missed by both patient and doctor. In these mild attacks, the symptoms may only be present for 2 or 3 days and be completely missed unless a rare complication like a small pulmonary embolus results from the unsuspected and unrecognized phlebitic attack. I have seen several instances of such small pulmonary emboli that had to be traced back to their phlebitic source. A careful history and examination will indicate that a small isolated area of tenderness and reddening had been present a week or 10 days prior to the pulmonary accident. The patient may have also noted some fever or chilliness at the time of onset of the phlebitis, and many of these minor attacks are undiagnosed and disregarded.

The converse is also true. The lack of clear understanding by many physicians of the nature of superficial phlebitis has resulted in many mistaken diagnoses for the following trivial conditions. Attacks of furunculosis, cellulitis, insect bites, contusions from trauma, or various types of dermatitis have confused physicians who are not experienced in the peripheral vascular field. It is important to avoid these incorrect diagnoses because the patient is often subjected to the erroneous treatment for phlebitis in general. This consists of hospitalizing the patient for 2 to 3 weeks, elevating the limb, and administering antibiotic and anticoagulant treatment.

Other problems in diagnosis arise when patients present themselves with a history of a previous attack of superficial phlebitis which was not confirmed at the time by competent medical opinion. Here, the operator must rely on the history of the patient, and it is often difficult to arrive at a conclusion based upon the patient's story. To assist in making a diagnosis of such a previous attack, which has since healed, the following prerequisites are listed:

1) The presence of an unhealed thrombus in a varicose vein on the lower limb;
2) Increased erythrocyte sedimentation rate (ESR).
3) A history of varicose veins with previous phlebitic attacks;
4) Positive reaction to a provocative test injection;
5) Positive Doppler test.

The best test is the provocative injection described below. If need be, the ESR will often give a clear indication of a phlebitic process. In my study reported in 1934 (25), the existence of thrombophlebitis in various kinds of varicose conditions was clearly indicated by a rapid rate of sedimentation. While I no longer employ this test as a routine measure, it is a useful confirmatory finding. In cases of doubt, sonic Doppler examination may be of material assistance.

Treatment

The existence of varicose veins, even in a simple form, is not the benign condition that many physicians and far too many patients believe it to be. Very often patients are advised to leave them alone if they have no symptoms. Doctors don't realize the dangers involved because these veins may already have a subclinical infection, or may develop a latent phlebitis if they are not treated.

It has been my long standing policy to advise treatment of any varicosities present on the lower extremities. After a medical lifetime of observing the crippling effects of varico-phlebitis, I have developed a healthy respect for this condition.

The treatment will be discussed in two parts: a) the older slow method of giving injections once a week for a varying period of one to three months or more; and b) the vastly improved rapid technique first described in 1961 (26, Biegeleisen), in which a case may be completed often in 3 to 6 days. Some cases may take 1 to 2 weeks. Only occasionally is more time needed.

Slow Method

The first injection should be the blandest solution available. This may be any of the following: 0.5 to 1 c.c. of 50% dextrose solution, 3 to 5 minims of invert sugar solution, 0.25 to 0.5 c.c. of varisol, or 3 to 4 minims of 20% sodium chloride solution (see Chapter 3). In very acute cases, it is best to do this first injection on the uninvolved leg. Occasionally, if the infection seems hyperactive, I try one or two vein punctures on the same or opposite side for initial study. If there is no reaction, I then proceed with an actual injection with any of the above weak sclerosing solutions. If the operator has a choice, he should make this test in the mid-leg region.

The reaction to this first treatment will be a guide for the balance of the case. In the normal non-phlebitic varicose vein there will usually be no reaction to the test injection. In the presence of latent or slumbering phlebitic infection, this first injection will act as a provocative test. A positive reaction is indicated by the development of an inflammatory response over the vein treated, which is usually accompanied by a small tender thrombus. This reaction may often be obtained within several hours to warn the operator of the presence of sub-clinical phlebitis.

If the patient exhibits acute thrombophlebitis at the outset, this test should also be performed as the reaction will indicate the degree of phlebitic activity present. Again, the reaction can be noticed after a few hours.

In the presence of active phlebitis, such a reaction, occurring soon after the test, may not stop at this point, if left alone, but could intensify by the next day or two. This fact must be understood in planning the ensuing injections.

The operator thus, with one treatment, has learned three things;

1) The presence or absence of any infection in the vein; or

2) The existence or absence of latent infection;

3) The degree of activity in a case where acute phlebitis is present at the outset.

In cases of doubt, the test treatment may be repeated at the same or higher dose using the same solution. Thus, sometimes one may not get a reaction with 0.5 to 1 c.c. of 50% glucose solution, but doubling the dose to 2 c.c. of dextrose might be more effective.

Before proceeding with the second injection, it is important to understand the nature of the *flare-up* reaction that occurs with this therapy. This is often accompanied by migration of the thrombosis in a characteristic fashion to further confirm the existence of phlebitis. During the treatment of these cases, and occurring with any injection after the second, a pronounced inflammatory response may suddenly result after an injection that has proven too strong for the phlebitic process that is present. This is called a *flare-up*.

It is identified by an incubation period of 5 to 10 days, and a tendency to migrate along the course of a vein. This is in contrast to the non-phlebitic response of an ordinary varicosity that does not migrate and appears from 1 to 3 days after a treatment. The injection method should be so gauged to avoid flare-ups. This calls for the careful technique which is being described.

Some degree of information will also have been obtained if the sedimentation rate has been taken at the outset of the case as discussed previously. The degree of infection in a latent or obviously active case is roughly proportional to the sedimentation time. I have substantiated this correlation many times, and it can be used as another guide in determining the treatment.

The second injection following the provocative one is also important because it, too, may produce a marked inflammatory result. Also, at this point, the problem of allergy enters into the treatment because one must remember that just as in non-phlebitic cases, allergic manifestations must also be kept in mind in treating phlebitis. This is fully described in Chapters 4 and 5.

In the absence of pronounced reaction, the operator can now introduce a few minims of the sclerosing solution he will favor in this case. The general rule to follow is that the weekly treatments must be planned in order to inject a gradually increasing series of sclerosing injections. Using Table I, which lists sclerosing solutions in the order of increasing sclerotic power, the physician selects appropriate medication for each case. It is possible to work with a single solution and achieve the same effect, provided the patient is not allergic to it and the operator knows how to control the degree of irritation by varying the concentration and quantity of the agent selected.

The second injection, therefore, could be 0.25 to 0.5 c.c. of sodium morrhuate 5% or a similar amount of 1% Sotradecol. The operator can dilute these reagents himself with distilled water if he wants to further reduce the degree of sclerosing activity.

At weekly intervals the treatments are now increased in potency, and several injections may not be given at one time. The rule is to produce the required sclerosing action with a minimum of inflammatory response. In the event that the response is greater than desired, it is advisable to repeat the same dose on the following visit. In this fashion, with careful control, it will be possible to move up to the strongest irritants, possbily after the fourth or fifth injection, without producing violent reactions. It seems that an immune state has been achieved so that the varicose phlebitis can now be treated with the same sclerosing agents as in the average case. Thus, full doses of Sotradecol or other potent irritants may now be used. In general, the same order of injections is followed as in Chapter 4.

In the event that the patient experiences a flare-up reaction to one of the injections in the series, this need not cause any concern. By prescribing phenylbutazone (Butazolidin) 100 mg. orally, using compression bandaging, and insisting on ambulation, these attacks should subside. The operator will find, after a flare-up reaction, that the patient has also achieved a state of immunity. It is now possible to use strong sclerosing solutions without producing any further flare-ups. Paradoxically, I have observed a curious fact that in the latter half of treatment, after achieving immunity, the veins require, in some instances, even stronger irritants than in normal cases. This is a further indication that the inflammatory responses in this therapy produce a special kind of immunity which protects them against further phlebitic reactions.

Rapid Method

The newer method of rapid treatment, which has been described in Chapter 5, is applicable to most cases of varicose phlebitis, with some modifications and exceptions. It is important to assess the degree of inflammation that is present before embarking on the treatment program. During this initial study, the operator can decide just how rapidly the case can be handled. Experience is needed for this technique which is not advised for the beginner.

The hyperacute case, especially with large bulky thromboses, obviously cannot be attacked immediately. It is advisable to administer anti-inflammatory drugs like phenylbutazone, use compression bandaging with ambulation, and abate the inflammation by these conservative means, before proceeding with the treatment. Temporizing in this fashion for several weeks, or even months if necessary, will convert the patient's phlebitis into a more moderate inflammatory condition which can then be dealt with by either the slow or rapid method, depending upon the operator's degree of skill and experience.

As in rapid method described previously (Chapter 5), the first injection is 0.5 to 1 c.c. of 50% dextrose solution. The reaction to this is to read after 4 hours and will be a guide for subsequent treatment. If there is no reaction the operator can proceed to injection number two which should be a larger dose of sugar solution. This can be 2 to 4 c.c. given on the same day as the test injection.

Two days later, if there has been little reaction, the physician can proceed with 0.25 to 0.5 c.c. sodium morrhuate or the same dose of 1% Sotradecol or similar solution. On this second day the patient may be seen two or three times with an interval of several hours between treatments. If there is no indication of allergy or marked inflammatory response, the doctor can double the dose of sclerosing agent by using 1 c.c. of sodium morrhuate or he may now introduce 3% Sotradecol, 1 c.c. At the end of the second day the patient will probably tolerate injections of 2 c.c. sodium morrhuate and 2 c.c. Sotradecol, treating small to medium sized veins on the leg preferably in the upright or standing position.

By using Table I, the operator can now select sclerosing solutions with increasing potency to continue with the treatment. It will be found that these injections, given after 2 day intervals, are less apt to induce violent inflammatory results or allergic reactions than with the slower method of treatment.

While the mechanism for these reactions is not yet clearly understood, it is a clinical fact that this more rapid type of therapy seems to overrun the body's defenses against increased inflammation of the varicose veins.

The object of the therapy is to safely induce mildly inflammatory responses in the veins to achieve the state of immunity mentioned above. This can be recognized when a full dose of the sclerosing agent produces a minimal thrombotic result as in the non-infected vein. It is then safe to proceed along regular lines as outlined in Chapter 5 to complete the case. The same order of injections is followed.

Empty-vein techniques are just as important here as in the standard rapid injection technique. Good compression in whatever form the operator devises, is equally vital to the success of the treatment. Gradient stockings and leotards, or various types of elastic bandages are used by some workers to maintain compression after treatment. There is no change in this area from the routine measures mentioned in the previous discussion of rapid injection technique.

I seldom use the slow weekly method of injection treatment for varicophlebitis. I find it useful for teaching purposes and recommend it to physicians who are learning the technique. The method chosen depends upon the physician. In both the slow and rapid methods, patients should be given a prescription of Butazolidin 100 mg. and instructed to take the medication with or after their meals in the event of larger inflammatory or painful reactions. Only a few patients find it necessary to take this medication.

The most important admonition is to strictly insist on ambulation during and after this treatment. Failure to follow this rule can be disastrous, and the patients must be so warned.

Both of these techniques, the slow and rapid method, should be aimed at producing the required sclerosing action with a minimum of inflammatory response. Ideally, the injection which closes a vein without any ensuing tenderness, is the perfect injection. This is difficult to obtain in actual practice because most patients will feel some soreness following treatment. Another reason for minimizing inflammatory responses is that, especially in phlebitis, excessive reactions affect the lymphatic vessels surrounding the veins. It is therefore important to eliminate phlebitis in any of its forms because persistent lymphangitis, which accompanies it, can be the onset of lymphedema with its undesirable symptoms.

Surgery for varicose phlebitis spreads the infection into the lymphatic circulation of the limb. Stripping procedures for varicose veins are often performed without taking into account the probability that latent infection may be present in the varicose veins. Avulsion of the saphenous system of veins, which interrupts numerous fine lymphatic channels, not only spreads the latent infection, but also interrupts the lymph flow and may produce lymphedema as a complication up to 20 years later. Injection treatment for varicose phlebitis removes the veins effectively with a minimum of lymphatic disturbance. Aside from the special techniques described here, the other features of treating varicosities by either slow or rapid methods remain the same and, to avoid repetition, have not been described here.

Complications

The complications of injection treatment in this condition are essentially the same as in non-phlebitic varicose veins, They occur largely in the treatment before immunity to injections is established. As described above, once the patient has become stabilized to sclerosing therapy, his reactions are the same as in simple varicose veins.

Extension into the deep system must be guarded against by avoiding potent irritation where communication with the deep system is present. Thus injection treatment of the perforator veins and the entry of the saphenous veins into the deep system must not be overtreated, so as to minimize extension. The operator must carefully calculate the amount of solution he is injecting to avoid a spillover into the deep system of veins. Effective compression is especially important at these points.

The frequency of pulmonary embolism following treatment has been highly exaggerated in the past. It is certainly less frequent than following surgery for this disease. I have only encountered five cases in 50 years of practicing this specialty. When it occurs, the treatment becomes a hospital procedure and is not within the scope of this book.

Lymph leg as a sequel to phlebitis, and its treatment is adequately described in Chapter 12. The injection treatment for phlebitis is aimed at the prevention of this complication.

Chapter 8

▪ VARICOSE ULCER OF THE LEG

In general, ulcers of the leg are due to venous or lymphatic insufficiency and, sometimes both conditions. They may be divided into two categories; varicose ulcer and ulcer due to lymphedema. The latter is described in Chapter 12.

A varicose ulcer is always a soft ulcer because the tissues surrounding the open sore are compressible. Its cause is primarily a retardation of superficial venous flow. Often there is a minor element of skin infection, but no other pathology is usually present.

It is most important to differentiate this from the ulceration accompanying lymphatic block. Often they are erroneously lumped together in the single category of varicose ulcer. However, the lymphatic type rests on a base of indurated tissue which may become densely fibrotic in character. Furthermore, while the surrounding area of a varicose ulcer is fairly normal in appearance, the contiguous epithelial tissues around the ulcer in lymphedema are often discolored and indurated. This is due to the retardation of capillary and lymphatic flow in their tissues.

The diagnosis is made readily by examination and palpation. The varicosities that are responsible can be seen on the affected limb and all but point to the ulceration. The skin opening is most often found at the internal malleolus, although it may develop at any point around and above the ankle.

The pain of varicose ulcer is always annoying and often excruciating. It results from the exposure of nerve endings in the ulcerated area. The pain is affected by the size of the opening, the degree of infection present, the amount of venous pressure, and the sensitivity of the patient. Sometimes a beginning, small ulcer may hurt more than an older, larger lesion. Older lesions are protected to some degree, by exudates which dry on the surface of the open tissues affording some relief from pain.

The pain in this leg ulcer can be relieved by any measure that reduces venous pressure at the ankle and relieves stasis in the area. In order to understand ulcer therapy one must have a clear concept of the disturbed venous flow.

Venous Flow in Varicose Veins

In the standing position, and to a lesser degree in sitting, the flow of venous blood, in cases of varicose veins, is either slow or reversed. McPheeter (27) demonstrated this by injecting Lipiodol and observing the flow of the globules of dye under the fluoroscope. It has long been accepted that this abnormal venous flow is responsible for the development of varicose ulcer and other pathologic lesions accompanying varicose veins.

There is nothing more injurious to the epithelial tissues than a reduced or reversed venous flow in the leg and foot. This in turn affects the capillary and lymphatic circulation of the skin and subcutaneous areas. Under these conditions, minor skin trauma cannot heal properly and ulceration takes place. Coupled with this is the fact that the highest venous pressure of the lower extremities is found at the ankle. Varicose ulcer, therefore, is more prone to occur here than in any other area of the lower limb. Treatment, to be effective, must be aimed at the restoration of normal venous circulation. In the absence of skin infection or constitutional diseases like diabetes, the correction of the abnormal venous flow is all that is required for rapid healing.

Conservative Treatment

Bedrest

If the history, physical examination, and laboratory findings do not reveal any abnormalities, the operator may proceed immediately to relieve the pain. It is sometimes advisable for quick relief, when injection treatment cannot be started, to have the patient rest in bed. In this position, with the leg flat or elevated, there is no back flow at the venous valves, and a fairly normal superficial circulation is established. The pain will be relieved quickly, and most varicose ulcers will tend to heal with simple bedrest. This relief is only temporary because the veins are not affected, and with resumption of the upright position, the ulcer will usually reopen.

Elastic Bandages

The most frequent method of relieving the pain temporarily is by the application of pressure bandages of various types. First, a soothing dressing with an appropriate ointment on a gauze pad is placed over the ulcer and held down by strips of adhesive tape or gauze bandages. A 4-inch elastic bandage is then applied, starting at the foot and ascending spirally up to the knee where it is held in place by metal clips or adhesive tape. The bandage is wound firmly around the ankle, and the tension is reduced as the operator ascends up to the knee area. The amount of tension that the doctor or nurse applies to the elastic bandage is guided by experience. If the saphenous vein in the thigh is incompetent visibly or by palpation or percussion, a second pressure bandage is wound around the upper limb beginning at the knee, again with diminishing tension as one proceeds upward to the groin area.

The patient is encouraged to be ambulatory, and the bandages may be removed at night for sleeping, but otherwise they must be worn continuously until injection treatment is started.

Pressure bandages for varicose ulcer are not curative for varicose veins and are used only for temporary relief. When injection treatment is administered, a different kind of bandaging will be required. Sometimes elastic stockings may be substituted for pressure bandages.

Patients who are wearing elastic bandages or stockings for temporary relief of varicose ulcer must walk to get effective relief. Walking propels the venous blood as the result of muscular contractions which alternately fill and empty the veins. This is known as the venous pump. In the normal individual, the blood is propelled upward in the superficial veins and then flows through the communicating veins into the deep system from which it is pumped upward into the pelvic veins.

This system will operate only if the venous valves are intact to prevent any backward flow. The blood will then flow naturally toward the heart. However, since the valves in varicose veins do not function, then the muscular activity of the leg cannot overcome the handicap of downward flow in large venous channels. Additional help is needed to maintain the venous flow in these limbs. This is provided by the elastic bandages or stockings described above.

Unna Paste Bandages (Unna Boot)

This old formula, which has a zinc-gelatin base, has been incorporated into a commercial guaze impregnated bandage.* It has been accepted by many practitioners for use in varicose ulcers as it is very soothing. It is especially useful where skin conditions result from irritant discharges in ulcer cases.

The soothing effect is due to the chemical combination, and it also acts like a pressure bandage to compress the varicose veins and assist the venous circulation. The gelatin in the chemical formulation absorbs the irritating products of the ulcer and provides great relief to those individuals who cannot tolerate the usual elastic bandages. These paste bandages must not be left on more than two or three days or the accumulation of secretions will undo their soothing action. They are sometimes kept on a little longer but should

*Unnacast, Medico Paste, Dome-Paste.

definitely be removed within five days. This treatment, also, is only a temporary measure until actual injection treatment for the varicosities can be started.

Sponge-Heart Treatment

For many years, the author has produced relief for stubborn varicose ulcers that do not respond to the above measures by the use of ordinary foam rubber. This is cut into various shapes and sizes to fit around ulcerated areas of the leg and foot. These local sponges act by flattening the blood vessels adjacent to the ulcer so that the process of walking produces a pumping action. This results from the elastic recoil of the rubber sponge acting like a heart by alternately contracting and expanding. The rubber sponge squeezes capillary and lymphatic channels intermittently, thereby producing a flow of blood through these channels into the ulcer area.

In addition to the sponges, appropriate ointment dressings on gauze squares will serve as an effective protection of the actual ulcer area while healing is taking place. This type of treatment will often work when other measures have failed. I sometimes put a sponge over a wider area which includes the open ulcer itself. This last measure is sometimes the difference between a lagging ulcer and a healing one. The pumping action here often stops the pain in a few hours.

Ointments and Antibiotics

These are of limited value in simple, uncomplicated varicose ulcers. One must not lose sight of a general rule in these cases, and that is, that a simple varicose ulcer should always heal rather quickly if the circulation is corrected. When this does not occur, one must look for other causes that are delaying healing. Often the practitioner will find some elements of infection which are interfering with normal tissue repair. It may be necessary to use antibiotic or antiseptic ointments or antibiotic powder to overcome infection.

If there is no infection, an ointment will still be necessary to protect the ulcer and keep the patient comfortable. I have rarely noted any difference in the healing of varicose ulcers that I could ascribe to the kind of medication in the ointment.

There are, however, some cases of varicose ulcers that will not heal in spite of correction of the circulation and antiseptic dressings. Here, one must look for some constitutional condition that may have been overlooked. This includes diabetes, advanced anemia, and possibly an unrecognized skin malignancy like basal cell epithelioma which is very rare here. The operator should also be watchful of ointments that are placed on open ulcers for a long time. Sometimes absorption of harmful medication may occur. These include boric acid, Chloromycetin, or Neomycin.

Some ulcers may respond better to medicated powder or calamine lotion if the skin is macerated or moist.

Injection Treatment

The conservative treatment of varicose ulcer has been outlined above in some detail. These measures are used only for relief of symptoms. To cure this condition, injection treatment of the varicose veins is necessary, as described in Chapters 4 and 5. This should be started as soon as possible because it will not only cure the veins, but also relieve the syptoms often at the very outset with the first few injections.

Temporizing with conservative methods should be used only when injection treatment is unavailable or contraindicated. Whenever possible the operator should institute a complete course of sclerotherapy. I have found that sponge-heart dressings and Unna cast boots can also be useful in conjunction with injection treatment of stubborn or advanced varicose ulcers. The operator must use his judgment in deciding their use in each case. In the end, sclerosing injections are the final answer to the problem of varicose ulcer.

Chapter 9

▪ VARICOSE VEINS IN PREGNANCY

The general tendency has been to accept varicose veins accompanying pregnancy as an almost normal complication that may well be left alone. Most practitioners treat this condition symptomatically and wait for the end of gestation to decide what to do. This inertia and conservativism is not supported by the evidence as there is a definite need for a modern, uniform approach to the problem of treatment.

Varicose veins may suddenly appear for the first time during pregnancy or, if they have been present, may become considerably enlarged. Previously, the reason for a conservative viewpoint was the fear of endangering or influencing the normal course of the pregnancy. In recent years, there has been the additional fear of sclerosing solutions influencing the development of the fetus. In my experience this has never occurred, and I have treated varicosis in pregnancy routinely. Furthermore, there is a normal regression of the varicose condition after term which favors conservative management. The last reason for not advising treatment is the tendency of the varicose condition to relapse with each succeeding pregnancy. For all of these reasons, most obstetricians have advised their patients not to undergo treatment during gestation.

The trauma of surgery did not influence this reasoning because many types of operations are conducted safely on the pregnant woman including surgical procedures on the uterus itself. Obviously, the aforementioned reasons were largely responsible for a hands-off policy in the past.

Suffering and disability are sequellae in many cases as a result of this attitude of temporizing. There has long been a need for a change in viewpoint as will be evident upon studying the problem of phlebitis in the pregnant state. While it resembles phlebitis in the non-gravid period, it has special features.

Phlebitis Complicating Pregnancy

The two general types of phlebitis complicating pregnancy are the superficial and the deep varieties. The differential diagnosis is most important because of the radical difference in treatment. The superficial type may involve apparently normal veins or varicosities. The deep type may involve the deep veins in the leg, thigh, or pelvis.

Superficial phlebitis which involves the saphenous vein or its branches often occurs in the latter months of pregnancy or the puerperal period. It is often preceded by varicose veins that are inflamed in a subdued or latent fashion. These veins may become the seat of thrombosis and so require treatment.

It is the thrombotic type rather than the obvious phlebitic inflammation that seems to exhibit more tendency to fragmentation and embolization, although this is not an invariable rule. In fact, it is still not known exactly why some cases of superficial phlebitis embolize while others don't. Nevertheless, the occurrence of this complication calls for treatment which will be described below.

Deep phlebitis in the well known form of *milk leg* is not completely understood. It may develop in the absence of any identifiable bacterial organism. It is considered an infection arising in one or two ways. In one form it may start in the parametrial plexus of veins and spread to the large vessels of the pelvis from which it may ascend into the abdomen or descend into the iliac or femoral veins. Another source is from the superficial veins from which the thrombophlebitis may spread into the deep system. Thus, varicose veins may become a starting point for a deep phlegmasia, a fact that has not been appreciated in the past. Sullivan (28), studying varicose veins in pregnancy, found that 50% of individuals with thrombophlebitis had preceding varicosities.

My reports (29) (30) discussed the frequent presence of latent phlebitis accompanying many cases of varicose veins emphasizing that the ensuing phlebitis is related to these untreated veins.

This latent phlebitis, if untreated, may become activated during pregnancy in several ways. First, the increased venous congestion may cause an acute attack during the last trimester of gestation. Second, the trauma and venous stasis of the actual delivery may precipitate an acute phlebitis. Lastly, the aroused infection may incubate and be delayed until the puerperal period when a fulminating *milk leg* may suddenly appear.

In the face of this knowledge, treatment of varicose veins during pregnancy becomes important prophylactically. This treatment works by a threefold mechanism. First, it removes actually infected or potentially infected veins which, of course, are a dangerous focus to leave untreated. Secondly, by improving the peripheral venous circulation it improves the stagnant venous flow. Therefore, it helps the deep system indirectly, tending to prevent deep thrombosis. Lastly, injection treatment increases the immunity mechanism of the patient to phlebitis, thereby reducing the threat of a spreading phlebitic infection. This action has been described in Chapter 7.

I have demonstrated, as far back as 1936 (31), that injections for varicose phlebitis serve to arrest the condition. The treatment acts by increasing the patient's immunity to her own infection. This has been demonstrated many times during the injection treatment of phlebitis accompanying pregnancy.

Latent Phlebitis in Pregnancy

In the phlebitic varicosity harboring an obvious or latent phlebitis, the reaction following the injection treatment is different from that obtained in the normal vein. In the phlebitic variety, there may be an incubation period prior to the vein reaction. These reactions have a tendency to migrate depending upon the severity of the infection and the strength of the sclerosing solution. With newer empty-vein techniques of injection, the reaction will be less bulky (Chapter 5). The important distinction is that, following a positive reaction to injection treatment, a special kind of immunity develops which prevents further *flare-ups* of the veins in that individual.

Once definite reactions have occurred, it becomes possible to use routine potent sclerosing solutions for the rest of the treatment. I have made it a practice not to attempt a complete cure of varicose veins in all cases of pregnancy. It is sufficient to prevent phlebitis from developing or spreading and make the patient comfortable. The normal regression following delivery will usually take care of many varicosities that remain. I usually limit treatment of gravid women up to the eighth month. Treatment up to and including the seventh month, however, often suffices for the average case.

Sclerotherapy in Pregnancy

Injection treatment for varicose veins in pregnancy has been pronounced clinically sound by other investigators. The following authors support this treatment rationale; Shank (32), Peyton and Loop (33), and Sullivan and Walske (34).

Hamilton, et al (35) treated 414 pregnant women with varicose veins by the injection method and had satisfactory results. There were no abortions, premature labors, lung emboli, postpartum phlebothrombosis, or thrombophlebitis in this group receiving active treatment. This coincides with my results.

Titus (36), as well as Adair and Steiglitz (37), also feel that treatment is advisable. Solomons (38) has written that pregnancy creates changes in the venous system making it important to arrest any development like late lymphedema that might become irreversible. He reported 450 cases with good results in close to 90% of his patients.

Surgery is seldom indicated for this condition because it adds an unnecesary shock for the pregnant woman. The treatment of varicose veins in pregnancy is in a special category because the degree of venous stasis is at its greatest at this time. It is important for the doctor who does this work either to have a previous background of treatment or special training in order to perform the therapy judiciously. I have found that the incidence of lymph leg is greater following surgery for varicose veins in the gravid patient because some degree of phlebitis may have been overlooked.

The most cogent reason for favoring injection treatment as against surgery for these women is the fact that with the best treatment available there is seldom a permanent cure of the varicose condition. This is especially true in the gravid state where recurrence is the rule for each succeeding pregnancy. I can see no sound reason for operative treatment here for this usually benign chronic disorder.

This viewpoint is not universal. Some workers prefer ligation and stripping while others favor surgery in the early stages followed by sclerotherapy for any remaining veins. Everyone agrees, however, that one should not aim for a complete cure in pregnancy because of the natural remission following delivery. It is almost impossible to completely arrest some cases during pregnancy because the varicose state is so highly advanced. Everyone agrees, therefore, not to aim for perfection.

The degree of discomfort present in pregnant women with varicose veins is often extreme. Obstetricians are familar with this. The relief afforded by eliminating the stagnant pools of blood in the lower extremities is well worth the time and trouble taken by both doctor and patient. Yet, obstetricians are often loath to recommend injections for their patients. As discussed previously, there has been an unfounded fear that sclerosing fluids may affect the pregnancy or fetus adversely. This is probably the reason most gravid patients with varicosities are left untreated.

I have mentioned previously that treatment should not be carried past the eighth month because it may take a month or longer for some of the larger veins to become absorbed or sclerosed following injection. The solutions and technique do not vary greatly from those employed in the non-gravid patient. Obviously, one should not use quinine and urethane as a sclerosing solution in pregnancy. The technique employed is similar to the one described in Chapter 5 with emphasis on effective compression. I do not favor weekly injections for these patients as this permits the development of allergic sensitization or phlebitic build up. The use of a modified rapid treatment plan reduces the possibility of either of these developments.

The solutions that can be used for these women include concentrated dextrose, hypertonic saline combinations with dextrose, sodium morrhuate in various concentrations, and Sotradecol.

A summary of the facts in numerical order follows:

1) Gravid women with varicose veins risk the development of superficial or deep phlebitis if not treated prior to delivery. Sclerotherapy tends to prevent these complications.

2) The fear of unfavorably influencing the development and delivery of the child by this treatment is unfounded.*

3) The treatment makes the patient more comfortable. Treatment may be carried through the eighth month of gestation and is aimed at relief rather than a complete cure.

4) Temporizing is hazardous because it increases the risk of a milk leg complication and the sequel of lymphedema.

5) Treatment is usually less hazardous than leaving it alone.

* Author's statistical experience.

Chapter 10

■ VARICOSE VEINS ACCOMPANYING ARTERIAL INSUFFICIENCY

Elsewhere in this book I made the general statement that there are few contraindications to the injection treatment of varicose veins. Now I must add that varicose veins can usually be treated no matter where they exist in the body.

The case of varicose veins accompanying atherosclerosis obliterans presents special features. The mere mention of injecting varicose veins in the presence of arterial disease of the lower extremities has evoked, in the past, incredulity on the part of physicians. This is understandable because the average doctor, thinking in terms of a lack of blood flow to the extremity, shrinks from sclerosing more bloodvessels. I have, therefore, found it necessary to explain that treating the varicosities assists the arterial flow indirectly.

The explanation is physiologic, and clinical experience bears it out. In this combined vascular picture there are two elements which interfere with normal blood flow. First, there is the narrowing of the branches in the arterial tree due to atheromatous placques, which reduces the volume of blood flowing in the extremities. Added to this, however, is venous stagnation or even reverse flow as a further impediment to circulation. It is a case where too little blood flow is further hindered by a slow return flow.

If either side of this disturbed cycle is improved, there should be an immediate acceleration of blood flow to relieve symptomology, such as claudication.

This improvement occurs even if the affected arteries are not treated. However, if the arterial side of the picture is also improved there is not only an initial boost in circulation, but a sustained improvement.

The most common form of arterial disease, the atherosclerotic type, is fortunately the one that most readily improves with careful sclerotherapy. I have not attempted it in Buerger's Disease or specific arterial conditions because more investigation is required here. On the other hand, vasomotor disturbances like Raynaud's Disease, acrocyanosis, or erythromalgia have not been considered as a barrier to injection treatment. The condition of livedoreticularis, which was considered a skin disease for many years, has been found recently to contain vascular overtones. It, too, will respond to injection treatment.

The treatment, therefore, is more or less limited to atherosclerosis obliterans (arteriosclerosis), especially in patients exhibiting intermittent claudication. For the multitude of patients with limited locomotion who cannot have surgery, there has been no such treatment in the past that they could turn to for relief. However, they must have varicose veins as a prerequisite for this therapy.

The degree of arterial impairment can be estimated clinically and by the physical findings that are present. There is a history of increasing difficulty in walking so that after a few months or years the patient finds he can walk less and less before cramping develops.

On examination these legs are characteristic in their dependent cyanosis. This may be intensified around one of the toes. On elevation of the limb, especially with gentle stroking centripitally, the foot and toes develop a pallor which does not return to normal quickly enough. The time factor involved in the return of the normal flesh color after elevation and then dependency is called the "circulatory compensation time." The faster the color returns, the better the arterial circulation. A time interval above 1½ minutes is abnormal and indicative of arterial disease.

Oscillometric tests, x-ray visualization with opaque fluids, and Doppler sonic estimation will confirm and measure the arterial impairment.

What the operator is looking for in these cases and, curiously enough, hoping for is the presence of varicose veins. Paradoxically,the presence of varicosities is a fortuitous finding because treatment of these varicosities will often give the patient a circulatory boost with immediate improvement. Some of these patients report the following day that they are walking better. This improved clinical picture continues as the varicosities are sclerosed.

Neither age nor sex is a barrier to this treatment. One must, however, look for the presence of diabetes which is not uncommon in this age group. If hyperglycemia is found, it must be corrected before instituting treatment.

The technique for treating varicose veins in these cases is different from that employed in comparatively normal individuals. I always begin with a test injection of a mild sclerosing solution like 0.5 to 1 c.c. of 50% dextrose solution. One should bear in mind that we are not aiming for a perfect cure of the varicose veins. The objective is merely to relieve the venous stagnation and assist the arterial blood flow. Since these individuals are practically all over 60 years of age, with many in the seventh and eighth decade of life, and with the added embarrassment of a restricted arterial flow, it is important to avoid major reactions. If the operator produces a massive reaction, it is possible to choke off all existing circulation because of arterial spasm. This could endanger the life of the limb. I, therefore, proceed cautiously from week to week, carefully noting the individual's reaction to treatment. The clinical improvement corresponds to the progress of the sclerosing therapy.

An actual increase in the pulse volume takes place. This can be measured and recorded on an oscillometric graph. The improvement is probably the result of arterial vasodilation.

Some delicate questions may present themselves during the course of treating these combined vascular problems. The operator may be faced with the dilemma of whether to treat an early case of impending localized gangrene in a toe or foot with this technique. Since this is not a primary treatment for the arterial disease, the answer will depend upon the judgment of the operator. Samuels (39), in his book describing the ambulant treatment of arterial diseases, records many years of successful conservative therapy by the use of intravenous injection in the arm of hypertonic saline 5% (100 to 200 c.c.). The prevailing school of thought is surgery of various types including bypass grafting and newer attacks on the arteries themselves. This subject cannot be discussed further here.

Vasodilator therapy however, should be utilized in these combined cases. Vasodilan tablets are often prescribed orally, and in selected cases I have cautiously injected vasodilators into the femoral artery for immediate arterial effect. These measures may add to the efficacy of the venous sclerotherapy. Tobacco in any form is forbidden as there is no known vasodilator that will effectively counteract the vasoconstrictor action of nicotine.

While the technique of injecting varicosities that accompany arterial impairment of the lower limbs is usually helpful, this method does not affect the atherosclerotic disease. It will merely produce a quick clinical improvement in many cases. It may even avert mild instances of local necrosis in the foot. The underlying pathology in the arterial wall remains unchecked and should, in all cases, receive appropriate treatment. I have, nevertheless, observed after varicose vein therapy clinical improvement lasting for years in those individuals who have the combined lesions of atherosclerosis accompanied by varicose veins in the lower extremity.

Chapter 11

▪ CHRONICITY OF VARICOSE VEINS

The chronicity of varicose veins was first reported in the *New York State Journal of Medicine* in 1953 (Biegeleisen, H.I.). One of the facts that led me to this conclusion was the frequent association of pes planus with varicose veins. This outstanding combination was never emphasized before.

No statistics are available on the frequency of this association except that in a 50-year experience, it has been unusual to find a patient exhibiting well-developed varicosities who does not simultaneously have flat feet. This combination is too high to be a coincidence.

In Chapter 15, I described a new clinical syndrome called *fascial weakness.* The genetic origins of weakness in the supporting structures of the body are described in detail and indicate that not only weak feet, but other sagging defects, are the result of an inborn deficiency of the fascial system of supporting tissues. The overpowering association of an inherited weakness like flat feet with a similar stretching of the vein walls led me to the conclusion that both conditions are related. Inasmuch as there is no treatment for flat feet, other than support, I was led to believe that varicose veins, a member of the fascial weakness family, might also be basically incurable. As noted in Chapter 15, the other members of this clinical group with weak fascial systems similarly cannot have the disease extirpated but only relieved.

While major improvements for the therapy of varicose veins have been made in the sclerosing solutions and also in surgical technique, relapses continue to plague practitioners who blame them on ineffective treatment or faulty surgical technique. Only a few seem to be aware of the fact that we are dealing with a chronic disease which is largely responsible for the relapses.

In order to understand how the state of confusion has arisen regarding the treatment of varicose veins, it is necessary to examine the early background of the treatment.

Background

With the introduction of sodium morrhuate for injection treatment in 1930, the cycle of modern sclerosing agents began. For ten years, newer and more efficient chemical fluids were developed. Sclerotherapy, the art of treatment with sclerosing injections, became an established procedure.

For these 10 years, injection treatment was widely accepted. About 1940, a movement toward ligation combined with injection treatment began. This lasted for 7 years when another swing of opinion became manifest. The reaction this time was away from injections and toward more radical surgery. Stripping operations were revived, and it was not long before excisions were once again advocated.

During the past 100 years the treatment for varicose veins has gone through two cycles of surgery and two of chemical sclerosis. It is clear that there is a continual shifting of opinions regarding therapy. My work, over a period of a half century, indicates that the chief reason for this confusing picture is the lack of appreciation of the cause for the disagreement. That is, the existence of chronicity resulting from the genetic foundation of the disease.

Other facts made me aware of the chronicity in this disorder years ago. Despite continual improvements in solutions and surgical technique, too many relapses occurred. Some observers attempted to ascribe these to recanalization. The author's observations over a period of years pointed to the fact that most of the recurrent varicosities were new dilations and comparatively few were recanalized veins. In other words, we are dealing with a vascular weakness of a persistent nature.

As previously noted, varicose veins is rarely seen in animals. It is apparently present only in humans. It is often accompanied by other manifestations of a sagging fascial nature such as hernia, hemorrhoids, varicocele, flat feet, pendulous breasts, and visceroptosis. In tracing the history of individuals with varicose veins, one is impressed with the frequency of these associated defects. As a matter of fact, the presence of varicose veins as a single entity is rather unusual. In 1940, I first called attention to this syndrome, which I termed fascial weakness and observations since then have straightened this conviction.

Relaxation of the fascia with accompanying weakness follows strong hereditary lines. Thus, a patient who has a hernia associated with varicose veins may come from a family in which one or both parents have suffered from hemorrhoids or flat feet. His brothers and sisters will often show similar familial manifestations.

In man's evolutionary ascent to the upright posture, the supporting tissues of his body have not adapted to this change. There are other exhibitions of of anatomic lack of adaptation to the upright position, notably in the inguinal canal regions. There, the muscular pattern and sphincter mechanisms are unable to meet the demands made upon them.

There has not been sufficient study of the tensile strength of fascia. This is an individual characteristic that explains the great variation in varicose vein development and other weaknesses. In clinical practice, patients with marked fascial weakness will develop recurrent varicosities quickly, following any form of therapy. This factor deserves strong consideration and apparently has gone unnoticed up to the present time. It should be obvious that an inherited weakness of this kind can never be eliminated by any mode of therapy and, indeed, experience bears this out.

Perforator Veins and Varicose Relapse Following Treatment

Varicose vein surgery in its present phase is unchanged except for the emphasis on perforator veins. Sherman, (40) who studied the anatomic distribution of the communicating vein system, suggested a technique for eradicating incompetent perforator vessels. This technique has started a new school of thought in the treatment of varicose veins. The theory is that recurrences are due to incompetent perforators. Sherman and his followers claim permanency with this new attack upon the varicosed venous system.

While the existence of communicating vein "blow-outs" have been known for a long time, Sherman found many more perforators than had been previously described and emphasized the importance of their erradication. He located the position of the normal communicating veins in the lower extremity and found them fairly constant in placement. He found five main groups as follows: (1) medical aspect of lower extremity, (2) lateral aspect of leg, (3) lateral aspect of foot, (4) short saphenous system, (5) muscular perforators in calf.

He did not point up the importance of the perforators in the Hunterian canal. He blamed recurrences on the lack of treatment for all these perforator vessels. He has evolved a massive, fairly thorough technique for dissecting out the entire communicating vein system. In conjunction with a high ligation, he removes all the perforator veins, claiming permanency of cure with this method. He admits that it may not be possible to find every perforator and also states that the perforators responsible for vulvar varicosities cannot be eradicated at all. He further states that perforators may have accessory perforators, which sometimes reroute the blood stream. It will be some time before an accurate appraisal can be made of Sherman's technique. While his method of treatment will produce relief in properly selected cases, it is only another type of partial cure. It is another method of treating symptoms and not the disease.

An x-ray technique can be used to locate the incompetent communicating veins. Masset and Ettinger in 1948 discovered, with their phlebographic method that communicating veins occur in pairs especially on the lateral side of the leg. They are often vena comites of a small artery, which they overshadow in size when they are dilated. These workers, who followed their x-ray studies by surgically excising the incompetent vessels, found even more perforators than Sherman and his school found. The students in this field state that the omission of any of the branches during the operation will cause failure. It seems clear that even with the aid of anatomic dissection, careful physical examinations, and phlebographic studies, some of these perforators will be missed. The zeal of the workers in rooting out the communicating vein system seems exaggerated. From a practical viewpoint, it is probably a hopeless task to eradicate completely this network of communications.

There is still controversy as to which incompetent veins play the more important role in the origin of varicose veins. Fegan (41) considers perforators as the basic cause, and almost disregards the great saphenous vein even if it is varicose. In pronounced cases of communicating vein incompetency, surgery has value for a limited period of time. Where these *blow-outs* are superficial and visible, they can be handled by simple injection treatment. More work is needed to properly evaluate communicating vein surgery in its relationship to the chronicity of varicose veins. The incidence of incompetency of the communicating system needs to be established because clinically *blow-outs* form a minor feature in many cases of varicose veins.

The relationship of the femoral vein to surface varicosities, when the valves of this deep vein are destroyed, is still an insoluble problem. This has a tremendous effect on varicose veins, leg enlargement, and chronicity. No effective operation has been devised to correct the condition. Deep ligation has been proposed but is, as yet, unsuccessful.*

There is no surgical operation that shows acceptable long-term statistical evidence that can claim a permanent cure in varicosis. Chronicity is finally becoming recognized as a characteristic of this disease. It is questionable whether the Sherman operation, or its modifications, will alter that picture in the future.

---

* Plastic surgical correction for valves of the deep veins is the latest direction of research.

Recognition of Chronicity

Chronicity has been recognized by other workers. Fields in 1950 stated that regardless of the method employed, no patient can be assured that his varicose veins will be permanently cured. His explanation of recurrences following surgery was that they were due to inadequate ligations or overlooked early new varicosities.

Three other reports concur on the viewpoint of chronicity. Kutz and Hendricks, who tried all methods of treating varicose veins, came to the conclusion that patients having varicose vein surgery should never be discharged as permanently cured.

Stalker believes that recurrent varicose veins are untreated varicosities and that the cure depends upon the proper operation selected to suit the patient.

Fenney in 1951 used an intraluminary stripper bilaterally on 89 patients and unilaterally on 117. His statistics, based on 1 to 2 year post-operative studies, indicated a considerable degree of recurrence, but he believed that beyond one year there was very little further change.

Nabatoff and Boyd agree that complete cures cannot be expected with any surgical operation. Lofgren (42) in 1974 writes that the varicose vein diathesis is an inherited, chronic, progressive, and degenerative process. He looks upon his surgical treatment as a control rather than a cure, and he is satisfied that a thorough operation provides an acceptable long-term result.

End Results of Surgery for Varicose Veins

Medical thinking about varicose veins must, therefore, be revised. In addition to the workers above who agree with my concept of a chronic disease, a leading editorial in the *Lancet* (43), summarized the British viewpoint independently arrived at, soon after my study in 1953. The editorial stated that "complete and permanent cure cannot yet be guaranteed in the surgical management of varicose veins." This viewpoint, while not challenged by present day British workers, is being de-emphasized with the advent of empty-vein techniques and compression sclerotherapy. The lesson of chronicity has as yet not been sufficiently impressed. It will bear repetition as modern workers in this field continue to blame relapses on faulty technique.

My series on the end results of surgery for varicose veins was reported in 1960 (44). It was based on a 28 year study of 200 cases. The material was chosen at random from private and clinical records in order to make the series representative of the results obtained by prevailing surgical practice. Since then I have refrained from further statistical reports because I found the complications and results have continued unchanged.

While other surgeons, as noted above, have issued post-operative reports on their 1 to 10 year studies to determine the percentages of *cures* none has stressed, or even noted, the disturbing complications I emphasized in my study.

Most of my cases were followed from 10 to 28 years. No comparable long-term study of the end results has been reported for injection treatment or surgery. The surgical procedures in this series were ligations, excisions, and stripping. Many of the patients had perforator surgery combined with the other procedures. A number of patients reported 2 to 3 repetitive operations that failed to cure the varicosities. The surgery was performed competently in leading hospitals.

Practically half (48.5%) of the surgical cases in this series developed a lymphedema within 10 to 20 years. This is an alarming complication for a simple disease, making the end result much worse than the original condition. Judged by this complication alone, the choice of surgery, especially avulsion by stripping, must be viewed with deep concern.

Of the 68 cases exhibiting unilateral lymph legs, 65 individuals had been operated on the same side. There were 29 cases showing bilateral lymph legs, and of these 24 had undergone bilateral vein surgery. This evidence confirms the direct relationship between vein surgery and lymphedema.

Twenty-nine patients had two operations, while 7 submitted to 3 operations. Some of these presented the worst recurrences. Some members of this group were persuaded not to have a fourth procedure, with great difficulty.

There were no satisfactory cures seen in any of the 200 cases in this study. Many of the patients showed a greater development of varicosities than had existed prior to surgery. The operative procedure had apparently spurred growth of new varicosities in this long-term study. Phlebitis in subacute, acute, or periphlebitic form, was seen on first examination, in 31 cases. Some exhibited fresh thromboses, others subsiding processes. Excessive development of capillary dilatations were listed in 35 cases. The complication of lymphedema obscured and prevented formation of telangiectasia or more would have been recorded. Thus, prior surgery did not cure or prevent the formation of capillary blemishes.

Many women had accepted surgery in the hope that it would give them normal looking limbs. They were openly disappointed with the capillary blemishes as well as the unsightly scarring. The latter result, in addition to the pigmented lymph areas, made many women deplore the fact that they had submitted to surgery.

Finally, of the 200 cases studied, 97 had developed lymph leg within 28 years. This is almost 50% and represents an overwhelmingly frequent complication. This practically irreversible condition, as noted above, raises a question regarding the justification of surgery for these patients, when an alternate comparatively harmless method is available for relief.

No surgeon has been able to collect this kind of a record for several reasons:

1) Patients do not usually return to the same surgeon in the event of an unsatisfactory outcome.

2) They usually go to another physician for relief and may have some complications at this time which are the result of the first procedure. This may not be recorded in the second surgeon's file.

3) Late sequellae, notably lymphedema, which often takes 10 to 20 years to develop, is seldom associated with the original operation. This may be completely forgotten or unnoticed by both doctor and patient. It is surprising because surgeons are generally aware of lymphedema of the arm that that often follows radical breast surgery with lymphatic damage in the axilla.

It is only in the files of an active sclerotherapy practice that cases with unsatisfactory results can be culled in this fashion. The files of the surgeon's office, or from surgical records in a hospital, will not show unfavorable results because the patients do not return. One must concede that if a perfect series comprising the records of all the cases who presented themselves for operation could be kept for 30 years, and if the patients could be persuaded to return for a competent check-up by experienced observers regularly for 30 years, we would have a more realistic appraisal.

In view of the fact that surgeons do not see their failures and that sclerotherapists are in a better position to study failures, statistics from either source will be contradictory. Nevertheless, the disturbing incidence of lymphedema as an overwhelming and frequent complication of surgery must be faced and considered before deciding on treatment. More statistical studies, of at least 20 years duration, are needed.

Injection Treatment

In assessing the value of sclerotherapy for varicose veins, one must appreciate the fact that scar tissue is formed as a result of the treatment. This is of two types. The first is a special kind of fibrosing reaction described by McPheeters which, if not recanalized, will go on to convert the vein into a fibrous cord. This subsequently shrinks as it undergoes phagocytosis and becomes a thin strand or disappears completely. The thrombi obtained in this reaction may be bulky and painful if proper compression is not applied and maintained.

The other kind of scarring is also within the vein and follows empty-vein techniques. Here there is adhesion between intimal lining walls which secure primary adhesion and fibrosis with minimal or no clotting. This is the preferred injection reaction and is followed by an immediate cord-like structure which again shrinks to disappear.

Both types of vein scarring which terminate in vein removal may sometimes be followed by the reappearance of new veins due to regrowth of satellite veins, venacomitae, or collaterals which abound in the tissues. They may enlarge in response to trauma of the venous system (in this case injection treatment or surgery).

The new growth of varicosities in susceptible individuals will vary depending upon the influence or extent of his genetic weakness. Thus, a patient with a minor degree of genetic deficiency who has a mild case not involving the major valves may not form new varicosities for an extended period of time whether he is treated by surgery or injection. This intermission may last so long that for all practical purposes this case would be classified as a cure. However, if the strain on this individual's venous system is increased by a change in occupation or other factors, new veins may suddenly appear once again.

Opinions will vary whether this is a cure. It is clear that more study is needed. There should be some way of measuring the inherent ability of the venous system in the lower extremity to withstand increases of venous pressure before becoming varicose. If such a study is done it will doubtless show that some individuals will never develop varicose veins while others will form recurrences regularly. This will depend on the degree of weakness of the venous wall.

With advanced cases exhibiting valvular incompetencies, especially in the perforator system, the degree of permanence following surgery or injection will depend upon various factors. One is as noted above, the degree of genetic weakness in the vein wall and the mode of therapy employed. The second is the location and size of the affected varicosities. A third factor is the degree of skill and efficiency of the operator who treats these cases by either method; and lastly, the firmness of the scar that is obtained.

The degree and duration of suppression of new veins in the disease will also vary with the stage of this disorder. Thus, I have found that mild cases, not necessarily involving the saphenous veins or perforator groups, may be sclerosed for many years (over 10) without any new development of dilated veins. Moderately advanced cases may be sclerosed successfully by injection without any recurrences for two to five years or more. However, during the annual check-ups any tendency to varicogenesis may be treated promptly.

There is another group of greatly advanced or neglected varicose cases in which not only is the saphenous system extremely dilated and incompetent, but the perforator veins are also involved. With the improvement is empty-vein techniques it is now possible to sclerose all the veins in these huge cases successfully, and by the use of compression bandages for several months, retard relapses satisfactorily.

Regrowth of Varicosities

Of the pathways available for venous shunts in cases of vascular injury or therapy two stand out. These are:

1) Actually existing anastomotic channels present in a dormant fashion. (Note: These are sometimes identifiable and anatomically known.)

2) Potential venous channels such as the thread-like satellite veins that often accompany large branches.

A third possible shunt is the delayed collateral circulation in the form of newly established small veins and capillaries which take some time to form. Though never properly studied in varicose veins, this process undoubtedly takes place. Formation of apparently new collaterals has been observed in occlusive arterial disease in man, and in experimental arterial occlusion in the dog. New capillaries have been observed to grow following injection of saline solution around the ring of old chronic ulcers (45). Uncertainty exists as to whether these vascular collaterals do not merely represent an opening of pre-existing but apparently completely closed channels.

Responsibility for the development of new varicosities following varicose vein treatment probably lies with enlargement of existing anastomoses or hypertrophy of dormant satellite veins.

In the event of trauma to the superficial or even the deep venous system, nature has provided the most intricate ramifications of venous circulation. Extensive secondary pathways are immediately available. Because of this, there is obviously never any shortage of venous channels. This factor, which protects the body in the event of trauma, prevents any perfect cure for varicose veins. Unfortunately, the venous system reacts to varicose therapy as it does to vein injury. Communicating and anastomotic changes begin immediately, and once again varicose veins may develop in this secondary circulation if the hereditary predisposition is strong enough.

Experienced operators report that after securing sclerosed palpable vessels, new varicosities may later appear near or alongside the original varicosities. This is clinical confirmation of the facts presented above. These are definitely enlargements of previously existing satellite or other veins and do not represent recanalizations.

Even if the major superficial system of veins theoretically could be eliminated from the lower extremity, this member would not be deprived of adequate venous circulation. There exists a complete venous system returning blood from the lower extremity through the true pelvis. This system collects blood from some of the tributaries in the posterior thighs and medical subgluteal region. The superior gluteal, the inferior gluteal, and the internal pudic are the three veins involved. The inferior gluteal may become enlarged and varicosed on the thigh posteriorly. The superficial tributaries of the superior gluteal may become varicosed in the same area. A connection of varicosities of the upper thigh may occur with varicose veins in the genital region by means of communications with the extrenal pedendal and other branches of the internal saphenous vein. Thus, there exists another system that returns blood from the lower extremity posteriorly through the true pelvis. It affords a venous stream or by-pass in cases of thrombosis involving the other main channels.

A refined surgical technique aiming at the elimination of a substantial portion of the venous tree only acts to spur this native venous instinct. Elimination of the major portion of the pathology is the best that can be hoped for. The maintenance of this result can only be obtained by the periodic control of new formations.

Varicogenesis, which will remain with the patient for a lifetime, can be held in check only by periodic treatment. A plan for check-up treatment in a typical case follows:

The patient's first check-up (following the initial course of treatment) should be in one year. Anyone indulging in this type of work must have an accurate check-up file to insure a strict check-up schedule. At this time, both limbs should be completely surveyed and any new varicosities treated.

The second check-up should be scheduled for one year later. Following the second check-up the frequency of treatment depends on the progress of the condition. On the average, yearly check-ups are advisable until signs of a slowing up of the varicogenesis is noted. When this point is reached, the period between check-ups may be extended to two, three, or five year periods. No patient should be discharged permanently unless a ten-year span without recurrences has taken place.

Conclusion

It is evident that varicose veins is a chronic disease and is part of a generalized fascial weakness which is genetic in nature. This cannot be eradicated by any known method, and can only be suppressed for a varying length of time depending on the treatment chosen.

Surgery carries with it irreparable damage to the lymphatic system and the spreading of phlebitic infection often in an indolent or latent form. Lymphedema, a practically irreversible condition in its later manifestations, complicates surgery as a late sequel, converting varicose veins into a pernicious and often incurable disease.

Sclerotherapy, properly performed, offers the best hope of suppressing the condition, providing periodic check-ups are performed. The problem is there is no training program yet available for teaching this specialty properly. This specialty has advanced to its present stage by the efforts of self-taught workers. The creation of training centers will advance this art so surgery will be reserved for cases that are not amenable to conservative injection therapy.

Chapter 12

▪ LYMPH LEG AND ULCERATION; UNILATERAL ENLARGEMENT

Lymph leg or lymphedema is a dreaded complication of varicose veins. It may arise in several ways, as will be discussed in this chapter. The epithelial, venous, and lymphatic systems are closely related, and infection beginning in one may ultimately affect all three. In the end, a lymph leg may develop, but this may occur so insidiously that the relationship to the original cause may have been obscured by time.

Extreme examples of lymph legs in the form of elephantiasis have been known as a tropical disorder since the beginning of the century. Here, the lymphatics are obstructed by a parasitic filarial agent to cause the extreme cases of massive enlargement known as elephantiasis. In other instances, the leg may become enlarged due to an hereditary disorder of the lymph vessels known as Milroy's disease. Also, gunshot wounds which become infected may serve as the starting point of an indolent, creeping infection of the vessels in the area which may eventuate years later in the form of a lymph leg. It doesn't matter where the infection starts; once the lymphatic vessels become involved, the ultimate result, perhaps years later, may be a lymph leg.

History

The knowledge of these relationships has been available since the work of Cruikshank (46), Halsted (47), Reichert (48), Homans (49), and Zollinger. These workers demonstrated the anatomy of the vessels and produced experimental lymphedema by artificially obstructing the lymphatic circulation. The latter workers reproduced lymphatic obstruction in the lower limbs of animals by inducing artifical phlebitis of the femoral veins. Other workers (50) produced lymphedema by direct chemical irritation of the large lymphatic channels of the lower extremities. It has, therefore, been clearly established that phlebitis which causes lymphatic infection will produce lymph stasis and the end result of tissue alteration known as lymphedema.

The lymphatic system was also studied by Castellani (51) who wrote in 1934, describing lymphedema changes resulting from cutaneous infection by an organism which he isolated and called Streptococcus (micrococcus), myceticus. The presence of this organism in lymph legs has not been confirmed by other workers. In fact, there is no known consistent bacterial infection that has ever been found in lymph legs.

The excellent research that was done to establish this concept did not advance until 1955 where Kinmonth et al (52) described lymphangiography using the patent blue dye method for injection and subsequent x-ray study.

With lymphangiography it has become possible to routinely study disturbances of the lymph flow in lymphatic disorders. This newer method of visualization confirms our concept regarding the anatomy of the lymphatic system.

Since the publication of Kinmonth's method in 1955, there has been a flood of reports on the extension and refinement of the vital dye method used to study the lymphatic vessels. Milroy's Disease (53) and numerous descriptions of lymphography techniques (54) are among the studies published. The injection of lymphatics in other areas has been the basis of numerous reports (55) (56). More recently, as the result of allergy to the blue dyes, methods have been developed for lymphography without them. Techniques have been devised in which the lymph trunks in the foot were exposed by skin incision, and then cannulated and injected with Lipiodol Ultra-Fluide. There is hardly an area in the human body which has not been investigated by this method of lymphatic exposure and identification.

Anatomy

The lymph circulation acts as a defensive mechanism against infection. Yet, it has practically no defense against injury to itself. It is an end circulation without the potential of repair except in a very limited way. Consequently, any injury is lasting and often irreversible.

Beginning in the intercellular tissue spaces where the lymph capillaries pick up tissue juices, to its final junction with the thoracic duct, the lymphatic system has a special arrangement. It consists of symmetrical, systematic distribution of gradually enlarging tubules, with valves to the larger vessels which are distributed in conformity with the arterial and venous ramifications of the other two blood systems.

At strategically located points, notably near the termination of the limbs, there exists a series of lymph nodes which act as filtering stations for the arrest of noxious elements picked up by the lymph vascular system. Also these natural filters serve for the development of lymphocytes and macrophages. The only inherent power this sytem has to repair itself lies in the potential of new growth in the form of collateral lymphatic capillary-size vessels. This process begins by vascular budding and has been observed microscopically.

The tissue of the lymphatic nodes responds to local injury by transforming reticular cells into macrophages. This is a limited attempt at regeneration and healing and usually produces ordinary scar tissue.. If not for this meager reparative power, any attack upon the lymph system would indeed be final and irreparable. Anyone attempting therapy in disease of the lymphatic circulation must take into account this extremely limited regenerative power as well as the terminal circulation that is present.

Etiology

Lymph stasis causing lymphedema may arise in several ways, since there are three systems that are intimately related.

Lymph leg may follow trauma which occurred several years previously as its progress is often very slow. In cases of this type, traces of infection have been left in the lymphatics to cause symptoms years after apparent healing of the original injury. War wounds are examples of this type of delayed edema.

Filariasis in which the lymphatics are attacked directly is another type of lymphatic disturbance. Here the lymph stasis is central as well as peripheral and the pathologic changes are consequently more widespread. In the congenital lymphatic disorders, such as Milroy's Disease and congenital lymphangiectatic edema (57), the lymph stasis is of another variety. Here the stagnation of lymph is dependent upon the abnormal development or congenital malformation of the lymph vascular system.

Lymphedema may complicate phlebitis in the lower extremities. Obvious painful phlebitis may precede the local lymphatic block. The condition may also arise from a latent phlebitis, to cause a lesion which is often termed idiopathic because the original starting condition has never been diagnosed. Sometimes a varicose ulcer which remains infected for a period of time may act as the starting point of lymphedema. In this type, the skin infection travels directly into the lymphatics without the intervention of the venous system.

The most frequent mode of origin follows stripping operations for varicose veins. This relationship is often unrecognized because of the time laps of 5 to 25 years between the original surgery and the late development of the lymph leg. This needs much more emphasis.

The complication may take place in an insidious fashion, sometimes with obvious phlebitis as an intermediate lesion but more often with covert or latent phlebitis that is undiagnosed.

Pathology

The pathology of lymphedema arising from varicose veins is the same as that of lymphedema coming from other causes. The phlebitic infection travels into the lymphatic satellite and sets up a mild lymphagitis. Thrombosis occurs resulting in lymph stagnation. The tissues become bathed by a high protein edema fluid. Drinker, Field, and Homas (58), in an experimental lymphedema, found the protein content to be 4%. In addition the tissues contain disintegrating cells. This is a good medium for the growth of connective tissue cells which is the next step in the cycle. The combination of infection, edema, and fibrosis, mitigates against the re-establishment of new lymph channels. As the process continues, the newly formed connective tissue increases and the fibrosis chokes off most of the circulation to the area. A cross section at this stage will show dilated capillaries and lymphatics, thrombosed vessels and enlarged tissue spaces.

Some of the capillaries rupture, scattering blood pigment throughout the tissues and causing most of the discoloration seen in these cases. The fibrous tissues increase and cause obvious hypertrophy of the subcutaneous layers. The collagen fibers laid down are not normal at first. They undergo mucoid degeneration and display abnormal branching types of connective tissue cells.

It is clear that this tissue becomes strangulated and is prone to necrosis which may cause ulceration. Once an ulcer is established in a lymphedema area, healing is obstinate and rarely occurs without medical intervention. The lymphedema process shows an inexorable tendency to advance. It does this by indolently creeping along the limb to include the entire circumference of it, or it may progress by sudden bursts of acute inflammatory activity which show a characteristic clinical picture. These flare-ups mystify many doctors who are unaware of the character of the latent infection present in all lymph legs.

The point is, that whatever the mode of progressive involvement, whether it be by ulceration, slow advancement at the margins, or acute flare-ups, the end result is always spreading of the lymphedema. If the condition is neglected, and advances sufficiently, the entire limb may become involved to cause a type of elephantiasis.

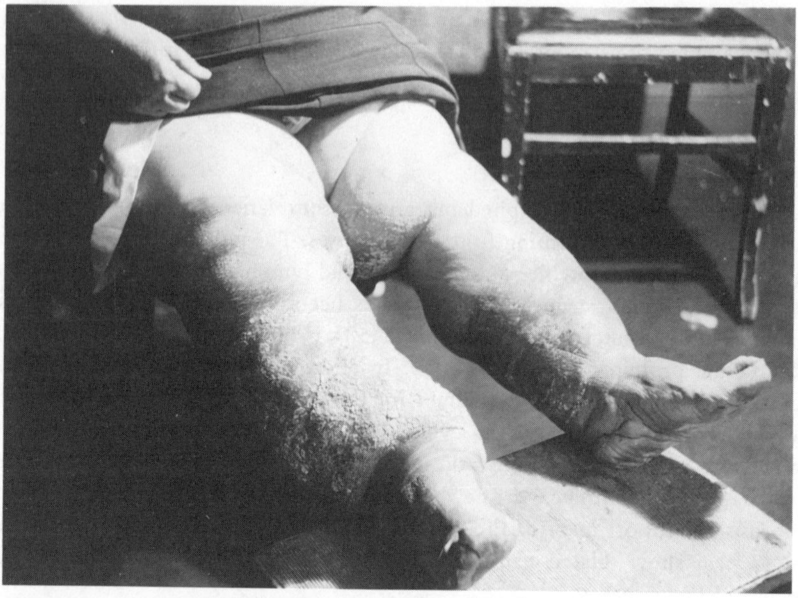

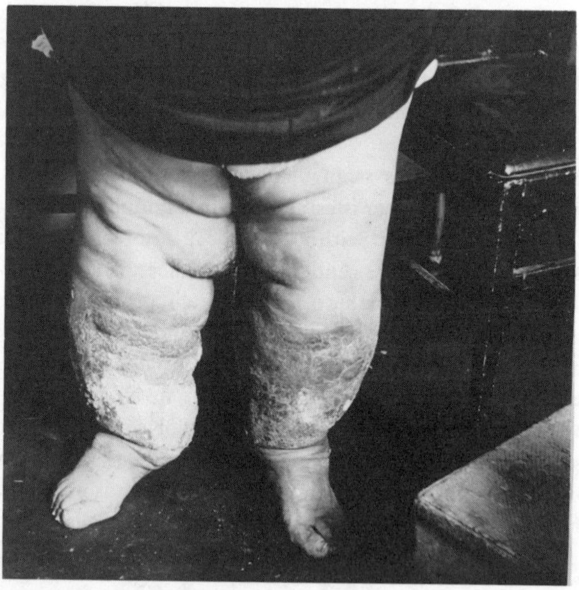

Figures 12 & 13. Pseudo-elephantiasis.

I have never seen elephantiasis described elsewhere in association with varicose veins. Here it is really widespread lymphedema which starts peripherally but advances centrally, staying above the fascia at all times. Castellani classified this type of enlargement as pseudo-elephantiasis in order to differentiate it from filariasis, a tropical parasitic infection. It is rather unusual to find lymphedema so widespread as to cause this massive enlargement. Figures 12 and 13 show the condition in a rare case of pseudo-elephantiasis with ulcerations.

Treatment

The name lymphedema describes only the first stage of this condition. The end stage is fibrosis. Beginning with a patch, often near the ankle, the condition may spread to cover the entire limb. Ulcerations developing in this hardened area form one of the most intractable lesions known to medicine. The principles of the treatment outlined below are applicable to lymph legs with and without ulceration.

Surgical treatment has a notoriously poor reputation going back to 1912 when Kondoleon devised the original mutilating operation. Torgerson (59) in 1931, noted that elephantiasis did not do well with the Kondoleon operation or its improvements. Kondoleon, himself, stated that his technique fails in cases of edema of long standing. In the original Kondoleon procedure, strips of fascia were excised longitudinally along the entire limb in order to relieve the obstructed lymphatic flow. For the enormous number of individuals who suffer from local lymphedema, nothing has been offered in the past except supportive bandages.

Injection Treatment

The technique reported by me in 1936 (60) had been used over 500 times successfully. Its principle is to open up the strangulated lymphatic and capillary circulation. This is done by injecting a special isotonic solution through a large bore needle into the lymphedema area by a special technique. Originally, a 21 gauge needle was used, but I noted that clinical improvement was more rapid with a larger size. I now frequently use a 13 gauge needle which is really a small cannula.

The technique is performed as follows: After local skin anesthesia, a large bore needle (13 to 17 gauge) is inserted from adjoining healthy tissue to pierce the involved lymphedema area (see Figure 14). If possible, it should traverse the diseased tissue and continue into the neighboring healthy tissue. This

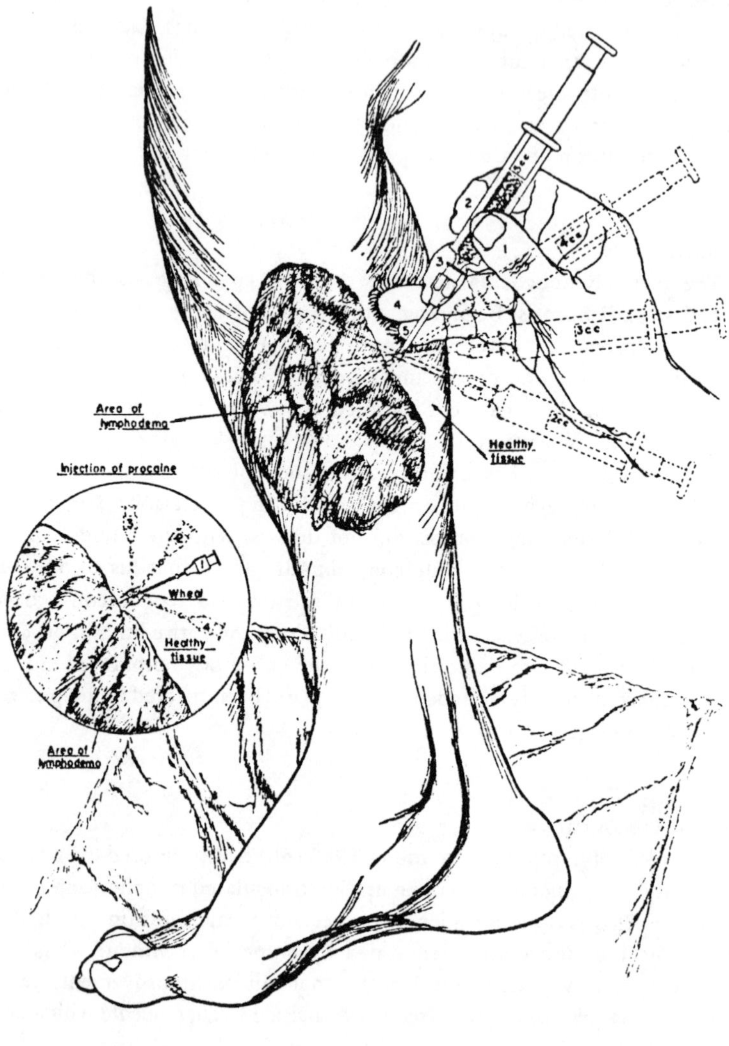

Figure 14. Injection treatment of lymph leg.

procedure not only connects healthy areas by a needle track, but also opens up the strangulated lymphatic and capillary circulation. The solution used, normal saline, is injected as the needle is advanced. The tissues, which are glued together by adhesions, sometimes crack audibly with the high pressure injection required. This further opens up pathways for new collateral circulation. One or more injections can be given at a time, possibly at weekly or monthly intervals.

Sometimes actual biopsy needles are used to core out canals in the hardened tissue. These can be of the Silverman or Biegeleisen type (see Figures 15, 16, 17, 18). If possible, some of the injections should penetrate the underlying fascia to further connect with normal circulation.

There are several isotonic solutions which can be employed for this technique; physiologic saline, Ringer's solution, and Locke's modification of the latter. The last one gave the best clinical results but saline solution performed so well in general that its routine use may be advocated.

The operator will learn that it is best to start the injection in a healthy area to avoid necrosis and to carry the needle right through the hardened subcutaneous tissue, if possible emerging on the opposite side of the lesion. If the area is not too wide, penetrating normal tissue first, followed by lymphedema tissue, and then emerging again into normal tissue, will give ideal results. This creates a connection between the capillaries in diseased tissue with those of healthy tissue on both sides of the lesion. These large bore injections must always be preceded by preliminary anesthesia using long 20 guage needles for this purpose.

Every case is an individual problem. The timing of the injection is important, and treatment must not be attempted during a flare-up episode. The operator must constantly be aware that he is dealing with a chronic lymphangitis that has a tendency to advance and spread. He must develop a clinical sense that will tell him when it is comparatively safe to render this treatment. This can only be learned by experience. If there is no sign of actual or impending lymphangitic activity, it is usually safe to inject. Considerable manual dexterity must be developed in order to place these needles in the proper tissue plane.

For this technique to be effective, the area of lymphedema must either rest upon a bed of comparatively healthy subcutaneous tissue, or else be surrounded by sufficient thickness of cellular tissue to tolerate the trauma of the large needle involved.

These conditions are not always present especially around the ankles. Lymphedema here must be assayed and treated with great care. It is usually impossible to find a bed of normal tissue underneath the lymph area at the ankles as many of these lesions rest on top of the periosteum. In these areas

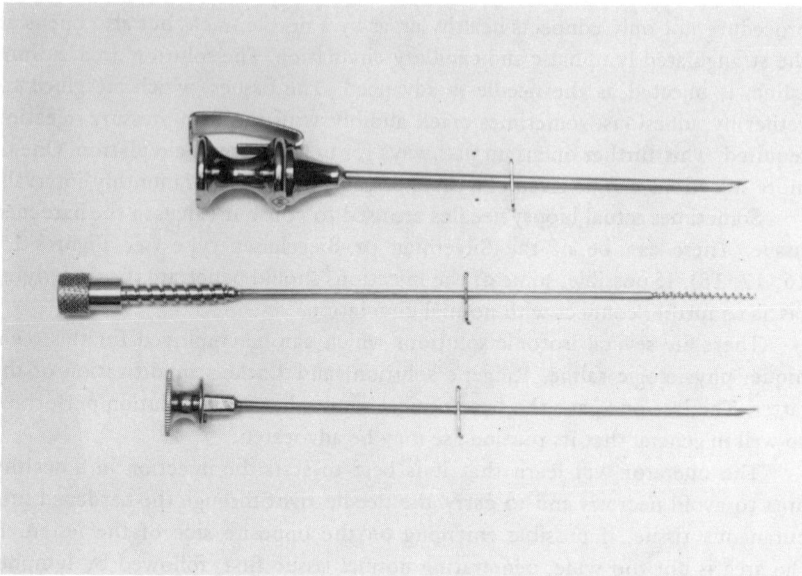

Figure 15. Author's biopsy needle (Vim-Biegeleisen) used for treatment of lymphedema.

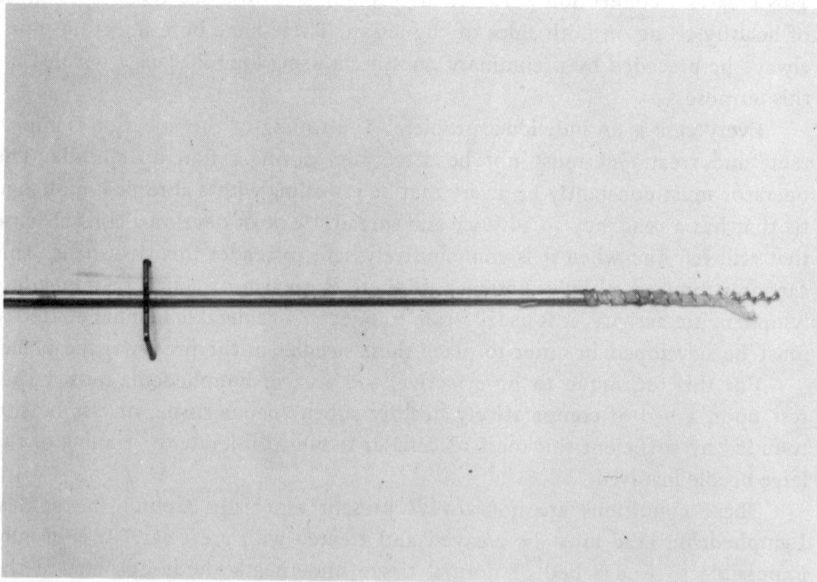

Figure 16. Author's needle – Note specimen in cutting grooves.

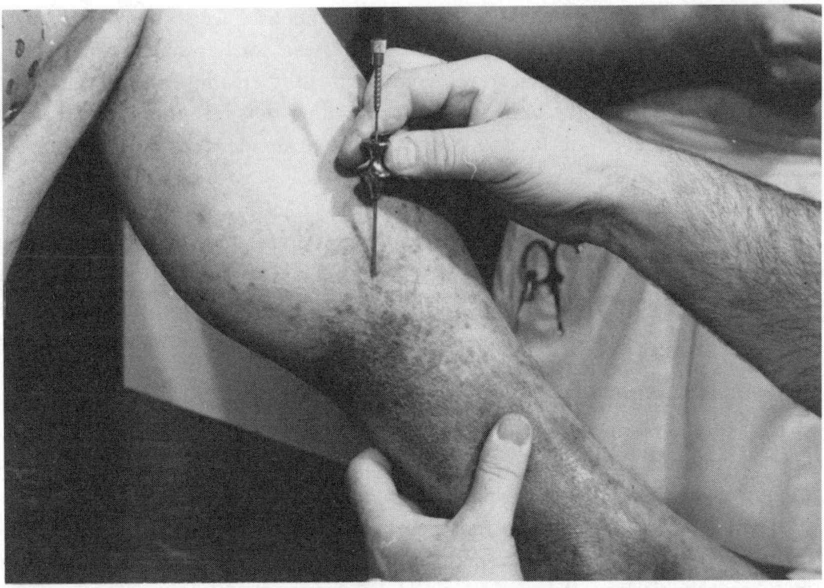

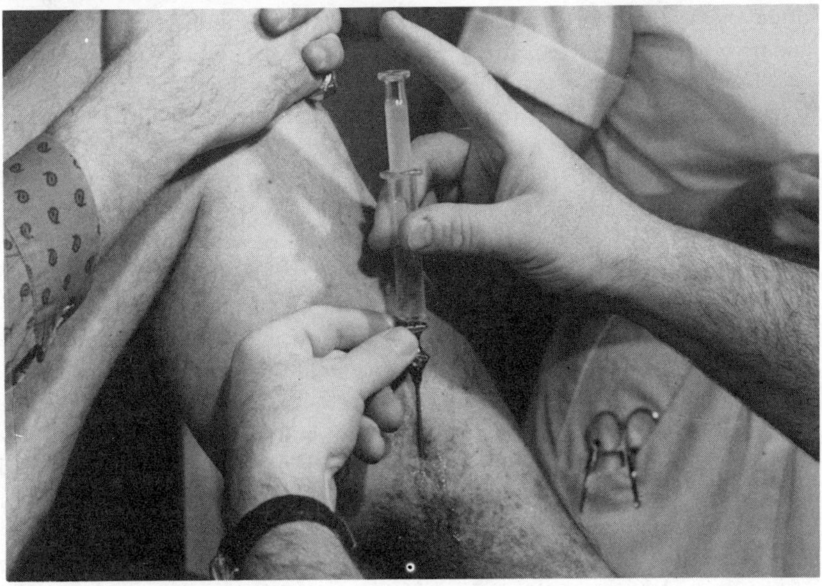

Figures 17 & 18. Injection treatment of lymph leg. Note isotonic injection after cutting cores of lymph tissue.

the operator must look for a lesion with sufficient adjacent tissue to tolerate the injection. Also, it may be necessary to use a smaller size lymph needle, such as a 15 to 17 gauge, to travel from the healthy area into the lymphedema so that an injection may be made. By proceeding thus, around the borders of the affected area, it will be possible to infiltrate an adequate portion or all of the lymphedema.

What we are attempting to do with these injections is to open up avenues of healing for the disturbed circulation. This therapy had its inspiration from a report published by Tunick in 1931 (61). This worker demonstrated that injections of saline around the ring of old chronic ulcers was followed by the formation of new capillaries. Based upon this finding, I attempted massive injections for lymph leg and its ulcerations.

This treatment works by boring actual channels which create tubular spaces, containing normal saline, that promote the development of new capillary circulation. The clinical results of this procedure are striking. In cases of lymphedema, whether peripheral or central, small or large, subjective improvement is noted after the first few treatments. Sometimes, just one treatment may be sufficient to stop the severe nagging pain that is often present in these chronic legs. It is frequently the only treatment that will relieve this pain even after medication and bedrest have failed. The lesions in these legs are often encased by encircling walls of induration that no antibiotic can penetrate and no other treatment can affect favorably.

The patients state that the affected leg feels lighter and more normal. In every case, in which the treatment has been consistently applied, the tissues become softer. The patient often calls attention to this fact since they had been advised that their affliction is incurable.

With the softening of the tissues, the color of the area becomes lighter. This is plainly perceived because, in extensive areas, the part that has been injected shows this lightening of color. Smaller lesions are completely cleared of the pigmentation. This, again, is a reversal of medical thinking which regarded the pigmentation of lymphedema as irreversible. It seems likely that the broken down red blood cells are phagocyted by leukocytes and removed. Furthermore, the connective tissue cells have been described in these cases as abnormal types with branching forms. These may disintegrate and similarly be removed by phagocytic action as mentioned previously. The parts treated become less tender, the leathery feel of the skin is lost, and the spreading of the lymphedematous process often stops.

The results obtained depend upon the amount of healthy fibrous tissue in the area, the size of the lesions, and the persistence of treatment. Small areas of lymphedema respond better. In the early stages, the condition may clear completely. In later stages, there is always a loss of pigmentation and the skin becomes softer and less tender. Some fibrosis may remain in widespread areas. Cosmetically, there is always definite improvement. Even in cases of massive lymphedema or pseudo-elephantiasis, persistent treatment will give a measure of relief.

Mention must be made of the findings in protracted and neglected cases of lymphedema. Some of these patients develop ossification of the lymphedema area. This may be extensive and resemble actual bony tissue to the extent of forming Haversian canals. The cause of this bony transformation is not clear but it represents an attempt to protect this area. A group of these cases were collected years ago. There is no known treatment for bone-forming lymphedema. Treating lymphedema early should prevent this complication.

Ulceration Accompanying Lymphedema

Any medical man with a flare for a contest will find the condition of lymph leg with ulcer an exciting challenge. This is a battle in which there are few rules. The expert pits his knowledge and experience against a vascular block accompanied by tenaciously persistent, chronic infection. Almost always, the physician will win out, provided he is resourceful and patient.

These legs crowd the surgical and chronic clinics of large hospitals everywhere. They are also seen in private practice. Called by various names such as chronic ulcer, callous ulcer, senile ulcer, and sometimes, erroneously, varicose ulcer, the victims make the rounds of hospitals and medical offices and all too frequently get no relief for their mutilating or disabling conditions. The onset may be shrouded in obscurity, often going back 15 to 20 years to a usually forgotten attack of post-operative or post-partum phlebitis.

Lymphedema with ulceration may arise from various other sources, but always ends up with a pathologic picture of lymphatic obstruction, and a special kind of fibrosis. Ulcers arising in this disturbed area are difficult to cure for one reason; lack of capillary and lymphatic circulation. The infection is almost always a minor portion of the disability. Relieving the obstruction will usually effect a cure. Healing is often astonishingly prompt, with few exceptions which will be noted later. Here is a situation in which the ingenuity of the operator is an important factor in the treatment, and his attack upon the problem becomes an exciting experience. The various methods of treatment will be listed. Many of these will be self explanatory; others will require explanation.

Methods of Treatment

1) Obliteration of complicating varicosities.
2) Vasodilating iontophoresis with Mecholyl.
3) Fascial injection treatment with large bore needles employing isotonic mixtures.
4) Bed rest with ulcer dressings.
5) Treatment of complicating arterial insufficiency.
6) Local application of antibiotic powders.
7) Application of autogenous clotted whole blood, as ulcer dressing.
8) Ointment dressings – antiseptic or antibiotic.
9) Spot quartz treatment.
10) X-ray therapy.
11) Vaccine treatments.
12) Adhesive strappings directly on ulcer tissue.
13) Compression therapy:
    a) Elastic bandages or elastic adhesive.
    b) Unna bandage.
    c) Rubber sponge therapy; prefabricated molded forms, dome-shaped or sponge-backed adhesive.
    d) Pneumatic boot therapy.
14) Ambulatory pinch-grafting of skin (autogenous).
15) Oscillating bed therapy.
16) Vitamin, hematinic, and endocrine therapy.
17) Local debridement.
18) Oral vasodilator therapy.
19) Wet dressings.
20) Silver nitrate treatment.
21) Tissue digestant therapy with Streptokinase and Deprosan Paste.
22) Porcine skin grafts.
23) Grafts with artificial skin. (see Chapter 27)

This is only a partial list of the medical contortions one is forced to exercise in the treatment of this pernicious disorder. It is apparent that it is no exaggeration to term this condition an intriguing challenge.

It has not escaped my attention that the use of antibiotics prophylactically or for treatment in these cases might be of value in their outcome. However, this has not been borne out in clinical practice, and is reserved mostly for evident, secondary infection requiring therapy.

The outstanding difficulty is the diffuse and almost complete vascular block in the area of lymphedema. On the surface it is difficult to conceive of the extent of this obstruction. Operative incision into this area discloses the nature of the problem. The area between the epidermis and the deep fascia is often converted into a hypertrophied layer of slippery fibrotic tissue, ranging in consistency from scar tissue to the hardness of tendon or cartilage. Only a Kocher clamp can grip this swollen layer of tissue effectively. One glance at this almost wooden tissue, often a half-inch thick or more, will make the observer wonder how the epidermis stays alive. It is this barrier to circulation that the physician must fight in order to produce any kind of tissue repair. It must be emphasized again that the clinical surface manifestation of ulceration, surrounded by induration, does not portend to any degree the nature of the obstructive pathology beneath the surface. Only experience with the needle can effectively gauge the degree of obstruction.

In addition, there is an unexplainable tissue lag in healing, the result of years of tissue starvation, which must often be overcome. This means that after the circulation has been restored the operator must stimulate devitalized epithelial cells which have lost the property of regeneration. The most effective way to quickly restore this healing power is by ambulatory pinch grafting. The response will often be astounding.

The treatment of lymph ulcer in spite of the prodigious number of healing measures is not haphazard. There are three definite patterns that may be outlined. First is the restoration of the circulation, second the control of infection, and last the stimulation of epithelial regeneration.

Massive surgery which aims at the complete removal of the strangulated subcutaneous layer is often doomed to failure because this chronic infection can never be completely eradicated. The amount of surgery done must be very carefully weighed against all the factors present. Similarly, the amount and timing of the needling procedures must also be evaluated clinically in order not to spread a condition which inherently tends to perpetuate itself.

The novice may be puzzled by episodes of recurring lymphangitis accompanied by constitutional symptoms occurring in the course of treatment. These may occur spontaneously without treatment and should not disrupt the treatment program which must be regulated around them.

In an experience of 50 years encompassing thousands of chronic ulcers both in clinics and private practice, I can remember less than a dozen which failed to close. These few cases either did not cooperate properly or were complicated by advanced arteriosclerosis which had been neglected. The outlook for the vast majority of ulcer cases accompanying lymphedema is favorable. Carcinomatous degeneration has been conspicuous by its absence.

Weeping Dermatitis Accompanying Lymph Ulcer

One of the most annoying complications of ulcer accompanying lymphedema is the presence of weeping dermatitis or, as it is sometimes termed, eczema. Applying ointments to this condition often exacerbates the discharging skin lesion, because not only do the ointments lack absorbing power, but they macerate the skin, adding insult to injury. Sometimes the macerations and the discharge further erode the already weakened tissues to produce actual tissue loss which becomes disfiguring and incapacitating. Extreme cases have been observed where the ensuing necrosis erodes the subcutaneous tissues to the bone. The most extreme and terrifying conditions may develop which sometimes suggest amputation of the limb as the only relief. It therefore becomes of the utmost importance to stop these weeping lesions early in the case before tragic consequences develop.

Paraffin sprays were used in the early days of this treatment. This was done by melting pure paraffin in a special double boiler, arranged so that it could be handheld, and the melted paraffin sprayed by a nozzle which directed it in much the same fashion as similar paraffin sprays were used in burn therapy. While the paraffin coating protected the skin surrounding the ulceration from erosion by the weeping lesion, it was found rather cumbersome as a routine method of treatment and reliance was placed on other methods of control. Since the tissues in these cases are denuded and exude tissue fluid, they belong to the same category as second and third degree burn cases, and burn therapy should be applied routinely. One of the more useful methods that is now favored is the use of artificial skin which provides quick relief and is replaced by true skin.

Tannic acid therapy proved a boon in the early days of this treatment as the solution formed a protective crusted coating over the denuded skin areas. The areas involved sometimes became blackened from the use of this reagent, but they remained dry and permitted healing to take place beneath the protective coating. It may be useful when other measures fail.

Another useful soothing preparation was plain Lassar's Paste without salicylic acid. This often turned out to be a gratefully cooling dressing which absorbed exudation and yet protected the skin surface. Sometimes sheets of special gelatin, such as Gelfoam, would act to dry up the secretions and soothe the leg. Whatever the method employed, it is most important to continue the vascular therapy, to promote healing while the tissues are protected.

Ambulatory Grafting

Since these individuals have often suffered for a considerable time, it is necessary to get quick relief. There are two methods of speeding up the reparative process; one is by bedrest for weeks at a time, and the other is ambulatory skin grafting.

If the patient will studiously stay in bed with appropriate nursing or sit on a chair with the affected leg elevated on another chair, healing will take place faster than with ambulation. This may require a rest of two to four weeks or even more.

Where it is not possible for the patient to be immobilized in this fashion, I have employed ambulatory skin grafting to assist the healing process with autogenous pinch grafts. Also porcine (62) or artificial skin (63) dressings (see Chapter 27), can be applied in the office. This is repeated every week or two until healing takes place. It is not generally appreciated how much can be accomplished with small scale skin grafting. Using a meticulous technique and appropriate mesh dressings, I have gradually grafted extensive areas of skin in a fractional manner to completely cover eroded areas surrounding an old ulcer. Even if some of the grafts do not grow in place permanently, the biologic stimulus resulting from the transposed epithelial tissues will act as a stimulant to rapidly grow new skin.

Mention must be made of the various other methods of stimulating skin repair. There are only a few true skin stimulants. One of these is the dye, Scarlet Red, in ointment form. This may be employed in strengths of 5 to 20% and is often successful. The best base to use is a water soluble one like aquaphor which can be removed simply with moist cotton. Futhermore, it is less likely to macerate the skin than petrolatum.

An equally good method of stimulating skin growth and ulcer healing is the patient's own whole blood. In doing the dressings, the operator will sometimes find that the lesion may bleed in some areas, This is to be encouraged, allowing the blood to clot and form a coating over the area. It will be found that blood itself is a spur to epithelial growth.

Iontophoresis (Cataphoresis)

A peculiarity of chronic ulceration is the development of so-called *healing lag*. It is as if the tissues are tired of fighting and are in an arrested stage of healing. No one knows why this occurs, but the fact is that a sudden stimulus will often start up the healing process and create a cure. One method of exciting indolent tissues is to abrade them physically. I sometimes scrape and nick the edges of old ulcerations, debriding them and causing the tissues to ooze and bleed a little. This will sometimes spur them to new activity. For a consistent method of stimulating chronic ulcers, one often has to employ the special electrotherapy of iontophoresis.

In this method, a galvanic current that can be supplied by one of several modalities is employed to carry a medication into the affected tissues. The solution employed is Mecholyl Bromide in 1000 to 5000 parts of water.

Mecholyl Bromide, an extremely hygroscopic and deliquescent powder, must be stored in an absolutely dry container like a cigar humidor prior to use. Once the stock solution is made, it can be kept for several weeks.

A square of white blotting paper, about 3 x 3 inches, is moistened with the Mecholyl solution. It is then placed on the skin above the ulcerated area and covered by a moist asbestos pad connected to the positive pole of a galvanic machine. It is kept in place by a short length of elastic bandage.

The foot of the same limb is placed in a foot bath of water containing a few grains of table salt with an electrode resting in the pan, which is connected with the negative pole of the galvanic machine. A current of 5 to 20 milliamperes is applied to the positive pole which is the blotting paper. Mecholyl ions from the blotting paper are carried into the tissues of the affected limb producing vasodilation. In addition to dilating the capillary and lymphatic blood vessels, the current also transports the products of congestion and inflammation out of the area, thereby softening the tissues. These non-specific actions are as important a spur to healing as much as the vasodilation.

When the current is first applied, only one to two milliamperes should be used until the patient no longer feels the needles-and-pins sensation. It is then safe to increase the current a little at a time up to the patient's tolerance. As the tissues warm up they become more conductive. The patient will tolerate more current, often accepting the full dose of 20 milliamperes. The treatment time is usually 30 minutes and may be given once or twice weekly.

Sometimes the blotting paper and electrode may be placed right over the ulcer itself for more effectual therapy. This method has proved uniformly successful in many years of application and will often succeed when everything else has failed.

Unilateral Enlargement,
X-ray Study of the Deep Venous System

Enlargement of one lower extremity has not been adequately studied. Prior to the development of phlebography, there was no recorded study. The first report, in 1939 (Biegeleisen, 64), describing a method for visualization of the deep venous system, was followed by an era of deep vein phlebography. This has yielded important results, but requires additional study for still unanswered questions.

With this technique the differential diagnosis of unilateral hypertrophy of the lower limb has been simplified. Other studies since then have established the value of this method, and it is now a routine examination for study of the deep femoral venous system.

Technique

The method consists of injecting a radio-opaque solution into the veins for the purpose of visualizing the venous tree. It throws clear shadows, even after dilution with blood, provided it remains relatively localized in the vascular channel.

A superficial vein on the leg is selected and 10 to 20 c.c. of solution is slowly injected, with the patient standing. Following this, a tourniquet is immediately applied above the knee, to obliterate the great saphenous and other superficial veins. The patient then lies down quickly and two plates are taken, after which the tourniquet is released.

The best Roentgenograms are obtained in the worst cases of venous enlargement. With a normal blood stream, moving rapidly, the dye is difficult to localize, and no shadows will be obtained unless the exposure is made during injection.

Three types of unilateral hypertrophy were studied:

1) Enlargement due to varicose veins.
2) Enlargement resulting from lymphatic block.
3) Enlargement following deep venous thrombosis.

Hypertrophy Due to Varicose Veins

Enlargement from varicose veins in the superficial venous system is well known. It is shown on x-ray in Figure (19). The veins in the opposite limb do not visualize, as they are normal and have a rapid circulation. Injection treatment of the leg with the varicosities results in a limb of normal size.

In the absence of visible varicosities, the simplest enlargement is due to dilatation of the perforator blood vessels. These are the origin of the *blowouts* which are suspected by a negative Trendelenburg Test.

This may be confirmed by the comparative tourniquet test of Mahorner and Ochsner (65). I rarely perform this diagnostic test because it adds nothing to the Trendelenburg reaction below the knee.

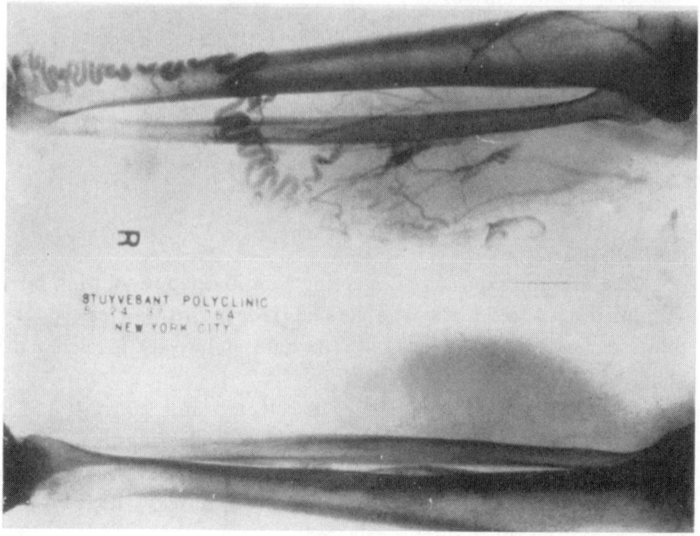

Figure 19. Right side exhibits uncomplicated varicose veins. The left side shows normal extremity and poor visualization.

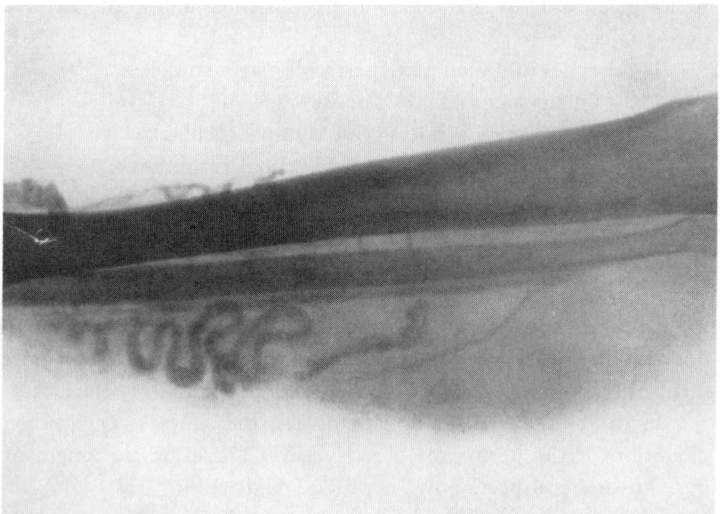

Figure 20. "Blow-out" or incompetent communicating vein. The other veins are normal.

These *blow-outs,* or localized bulges, spring back after finger pressure. This sensation is usually enough to diagnose the presence of an incompetent communicating vein. Figure (20) shows such a case with the deep system normally visualized. The leg hypertrophy is clearly due to the enlarged communicating veins. However, these enlarged communicators are not always seen on the surface, and may cause a confusing hypertrophy which can be demonstrated radiographically.

Enlargement as a Result of Lymphatic Block

Chronic lymph stasis may arise from a variety of causes as discussed previously. The pathology of chronic lymphangitis is present in all of these cases. It may take years for enough obstruction to take place before symptoms of enlargement develop. When this condition is in an early phase, it is often misdiagnosed.

The kind of lymph block that is found may be peripheral or central. The peripheral type develops as a hard, non-pitting local edema with pigmentation or other skin changes. In the central type, the entire extremity is affected.

The central type sometimes follows post-partum milk leg. The peripheral type occurs with infection above the fascia, as in the case of wounds, skin infections, or phlebitis of superficial veins. Skin changes occur most readily in the localized peripheral types, but cases starting centrally may develop changes in the subcutaneous tissues peripherally. Ulcerations may occur. Figure (21) shows a case of extensive lymphedema and a few superficial varicosities. The tibial and popliteal veins are normal, excluding the diagnosis of deep thrombosis.

Enlargement Following Deep Venous Thrombosis

The condition of deep venous thrombosis may cause permanent swelling of the lower extremity for which no treatment is, as yet available. It has been held for years that the enlargement in these cases was the result of a deep venous block. Perthes devised a special test that was intended to aid in the diagnosis. In this test, the great saphenous vein was obliterated by tightening a tourniquet above the knee. The patient was then instructed to walk briskly. It was accepted that any increase in size of the superficial venous system was an indication of deep venous block. Injection treatment was contraindicated in the presence of superficial varicosities. This test is rarely performed due to the absence of positive reactions. I was led, by my own negative findings, to suspect the existence

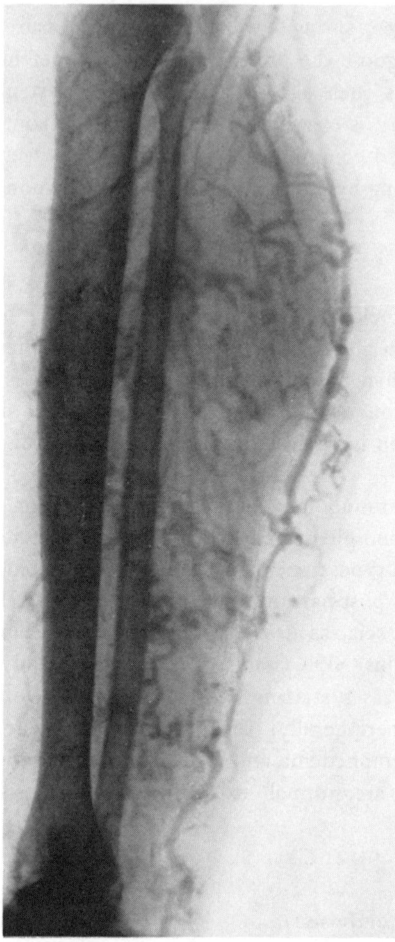

Fig. 21

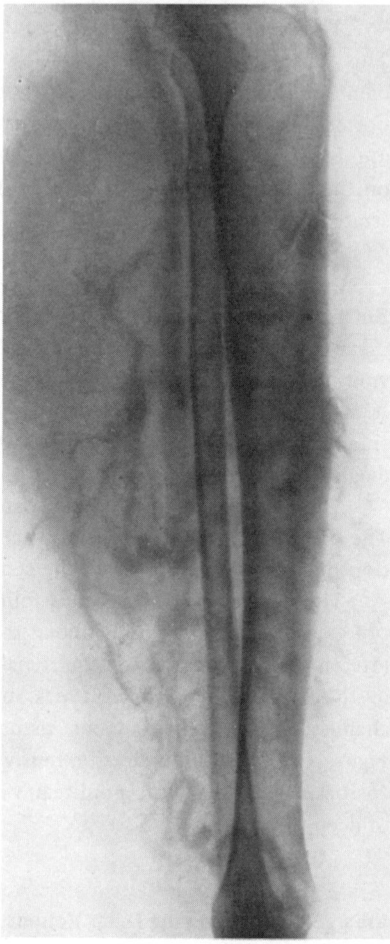

Fig. 22

Figure 21. Enlargement from extensive lymphedema and a few superficial varicosities. There is no deep thrombosis now.

Figure 22. Enlargement due to post-partum phlebitis with an extensive deep collateral network.

of a fairly adequate deep circulation. Radiographic contrast studies of such hypertrophied limbs, following deep venous thrombosis, were instituted.

Figure (22) shows a case of enlargement following post-partum phlebitis. There is a decrease in the size of the tibial and popliteal vessels. The x-ray shows an extensive deep collateral network. There is no evidence of a deep venous block, merely a relative one, with an adequate venous return.

The question of what takes place after deep femoral thrombosis requires further study. In some of these cases the deep veins may heal almost normally so that there is no immediate or long-term complication. In others, the valves in the deep veins may be damaged, creating incompetency of the deep venous system. There is, as yet, no remedy for this development as it causes permanent damage to the venous circulation.

In a third group of cases, the infection travels into the lymphatics, which accompany the veins, and slowly produces the familiar picture of peripheral or central lymph block, with all the attendant sequelae described previously. This may take a few years or as much as 20 to 30 years to develop.

Most authorities agree that varicose veins accompanying unilateral limb enlargement should be treated. This is best done by compression sclerotherapy after the patient has worn a gradient pressure elastic support to restore the venous pump in the affected leg. There is no known treatment for incompetency of the deep veins, although the latest research is in the direction of replacing the damaged valves by new ones.

Chapter 13

▪ CAPILLARY DILATATIONS AND THEIR TREATMENT

Dilatations of the capillaries are termed telangiectasia. They are seen frequently in association with varicose veins but they may exist as a separate condition in the absence of varicosities. When I originally published my report in 1934 (66), describing a micro-injection technique, there had been no satisfactory treatment for this unsightly vascular blemish. My original technique and the recommended solutions have been substantially unchanged for almost 50 years, a tribute to their successful use.

Generalized capillary dilatation does occur in other conditions, and telangiectasia of the lower limbs must be differentiated from these. The dilated capillaries on the lower extremities seldom project above the skin surface. They belong to the group of secondary telangiectasia, in accord with Madden's (67) classification.

The dilated vessels take various shapes from a straight line to the complicated spider web patterns that are often seen. They may vary in color from pinkish to dark red or dark blue. They are seen in greatest numbers between the ages of 20 and 40 years, and more frequently in women than in men. These capillary loops seldom develop thrombi.

Cosmetically poor or ineffective methods of therapy were formerly employed in the treatment of these lesions. Included among these were cautery, surgical galvanism, multiple linear scarification, radium therapy, radiotherapy, electrodessication, and CO_2 snow. Since all these methods involve the production of more or less scar tissue, they inevitably give poor cosmetic results. These dilated capillaries are often present in straight lines, several inches long. Skin destroying agents, in these cases, would cause widespread scar formation. Therefore, some investigators attempted to eradicate these lesions by the use of subcutaneous, perivascular injections of irritating substances. I also investigated these perivascular sclerosing techniques more thoroughly, hoping that improved cosmetic results could be obtained in this fashion.

It was felt that if the subcutaneous injection of a harmless sclerosing solution could remove dilated capillaries, this would offer the simplest method of treatment. Before other types of therapy were considered, therefore, a thorough testing of this technique was made using 17 different solutions (68). However, no change occurred in the telangiectatic capillaries, in spite of the marked induration and fibrotic contractions which were obtained.

Similar results were seen with the other solutions employed. Although occasionally fibrosis was produced, no improvements in the capillary blemishes resulted. In addition, no case of capillary thrombosis was seen after the use of any of the 17 solutions. The subcutaneous mode of treatment seemed to be a complete failure.

It was evident, at this point, that in order to remove dilated capillaries, it was necessary to bring sclerosing fluid into direct contact with endothelium. Obviously, intravascular injections of the tiny vessels would have to be made. Ordinary methods of injection would not suffice for these tiny vessels. I, therefore, devised a new and finer technique which is described below.

Micro-Injection Technique

The necessary equipment for this method includes: a) proper illumination, b) an adequate binocular loupe, c) special solutions, and d) special fine needles.

Illumination

The lighting must be of the operating room type and mobile. I found a movable floor lamp (Castle) with a shadow-free light ideal for this purpose. It is also possible to use an overhead operating light which can be directed to any area under treatment. However, the head of the operator will often interfere with good illumination, and I prefer the floor lamp type. It is also possible to have the operating light fastened to a convenient wall bracket so that the light beam can be directed and moved on the patient's lower extremities. A superior type of light combined with magnification is the modern operating microscope which is also used for eye and ear work. However, it is not practical to cover the entire lower extremity with this kind of bulky, slow moving equipment. Since numerous multiple injections are needed, it has limited value. Where the operator desires to clear a specific area containing especially fine capillary vessels, it might be expedient to employ the operating microscope. From a practical point of view, the mobile floor lamp is still the most practical answer to the lighting problem.

Magnification

A good binocular loupe is needed for this part of the equipment. I have tried every binocular loupe available in this country. Only a few have been acceptable, as it is necessary to obtain a magnification of 3x and still get a working distance of 9 to 12 inches between the lenses and the skin of the patient. I prefer an instrument that is imported from several European countries who make a special jeweler's loupe which I find suitable for this injection technique. However, there are many variations made in this country, some of which can be attached to eyeglasses and headbands that are satisfactory to some operators. The important goal is a 9 to 12 inch working distance and a good magnification that will be acceptable to the therapist. In this country custom-made binocular loupes (surgical telescopes) are available, made by Morrel Instruments.* These may be fitted to the operator.

Solutions

My original description of sodium chloride with an anesthetic in distilled water is still, in my opinion, the best solution for capillary work. I find a 23% concentration useful for most of the lower extremities reserving 21 or 25% for special indications. For instance, the 21% should be used in the ankle area where the skin is especially sensitive, and 25% sometimes has to be employed in cases where the 23% is ineffective. For the past number of years, a European solution, which has been mentioned in Chapter 3, has a special use in capillary work. This medication, called Aethoxysklerol, comes in the following strengths: 0.5, 1, 2, and 4%. The 0.5% and 1% may sometimes be injected subcutaneously without entering a blood vessel and sclerose a capillary without causing necrosis. Apparently it goes through the capillary wall to enter its lumen. It is used intravascularly in the 1 or 2% concentration for these injections. Aethoxysklerol produces more skin pigmentation than the salt solutions which I prefer. Aethoxysklerol is now available in aqueous solution.

Needles

Needles are a special subject because they have been commercially unobtainable in the finest sizes needed for this minute delicate work. While 30 and 31 gauges may sometimes be obtained from the usual surgical suppliers, they have a somewhat limited use in capillary work. Needles that are smaller than this must be specially made. I routinely employ a handmade, 32 and 33 gauge needle with a sharp tip that is 5/16 to 6/16 inches in length. This is used for the finest injections.

---

*Morrell Instrument Co., Syosset N.Y.

In order to locate and mark the capillary network, the patient must stand on a table. I use an ordinary ball-point pen for this purpose. This is necessary because, on lying down for the treatment, it may not be possible to find the smallest capillaries that show clearly in the upright position.

When magnified by a binocular loupe, the blood vessels under treatment will stand out clearly. These are either capillaries, capillary venules, or arterial capillaries. Since they are difficult to differentiate, even with magnification, no attempt was made to distinguish between the various types. As has been described previously, the tissue surrounding the dilated capillaries are of great density. The highly cellular epidermis with its papillary projections lies above and to the side of the tiny blood vessels. Below lies another dense structure composed of interlacing fibrous and elastic tissue fibers. Thus, the tiny vessels cannot roll away from the needle point since they are held firmly in place. With proper technique, they are transfixed with comparative ease.

Healthy tissue should be the starting point for injection. The fine needle point is kept near the skin surface so it will engage the vessel directly beneath the epidermis, and then is carried toward the offending capillary, bevel up. A gentle but firm push should enable one to catch the needle point in the capillary wall and penetrate to the lumen. Although delicate, the procedure is not difficult. Often entry into capillaries of smaller diameter than the needle itself can be made due to the elasticity of the vessel.

With successful engagement of the needle in the capillary, rapid injection of the fluid is made, making the vessel swell visibly. As it displaces the blood in the telangiectatic tubules, the sclerosing fluid can usually be seen. One must observe care to avoid perivascular injection. This occurrence will be demonstrated by the formation of a wheal, and injection should be stopped immediately in order to avoid a slough.

Quinine solution cannot be used because it often produces dark pigmentation which is more unsightly than the original telangiectasis. A 2 to 5% sodium morrhuate solution may be attempted, with caution, since it is not only capable of slough formation but also pigmentation (69). Any of the other mild sclerosing agents are also suitable for this technique.

An almost magical disappearance of the capillary groups follows successful treatment in most cases. Spider web formations, or connected clusters of capillaries, respond especially well to this therapy. Thromboses will be visible in many cases as firm green or dark stripes corresponding to the pattern of the blood vessels injected. These are clearly noticeable through the thin skin and are slowly but definitely absorbed within a few weeks time. The final result, after proper treatment, is a definite, clean, scarless removal of the offending capillaries.

Complications

There are two complications that may occur with this treatment; skin necrosis and pigmentation. Sloughing of the superficial skin may occur after perivascular injection of sufficient sclerosing solution. Around the ankles, where the venous pressure is at its maximum and stasis may be severe, sloughing can occur even with perfect technique if strong solutions are used. For this reason, I always recommend a 20 or 21% solution of sodium chloride in this area to avoid necrosis. These weaker solutions will successfully sclerose the capillaries in the ankle and foot area, while they might be ineffective higher up.

A hint of possible necrosis will be obtained during the injection treatment by excessive and prolonged redness of the area following treatment. If this occurs, an icepack applied may relieve the congestion and assist in preventing a slough. I usually flood the area immediately with 1% Procaine solution and follow this sometimes with normal saline to wash out any exudate containing traces of the sclerosing fluid. This often prevents necrosis. The most common warning of possible sloughing is whealing, which is a strong warning signal to stop the injection. It will also be noted that the fluid is not entering the blood vessel and coursing through its canal. Flooding with Procaine should promptly follow as noted above.

If a slough develops, it is usually preceded by a skin blister which is like any other blister and should be treated the same way. Sometimes these blisters will be absorbed, but if the skin erodes, the underlying raw area must be dressed for several weeks or months to keep it sterile while healing takes place. Sloughs always heal in the end, but patients need to be supervised and encouraged. In general they are treated like sloughs following varicose vein injections described in Chapter 6.

Pigmentation may occur in susceptible individuals, especially brunettes or others who have a high degree of melanin in their epidermal tissues. This cosmetically undesirable occurrence is usually trivial and will often fade by itself within a year or two if left alone. In the event the patient is anxious for cosmetic improvement, this may be afforded by special bleach formulae. The most effective one, in my experience, is an ointment called Solaquin Forte, 4%*. This must be applied and rubbed in gently for one to three months, and it will often lighten or remove the pigment stain.

The condition of blotches on the lower extremities is an annoying red to purple discoloration that is difficult to classify. They can usually be blanched

---

* Elder Company

by pressure, unless they extend into the subcutaneous tissues which gives them the character of angiomas and makes them more difficult to treat. When they are fed by enlarged capillaries the usual injections as described above may remove part or all of the lesion. Treatment is discussed in greater detail in the next chapter.*

Results

Mild cases of telangiectasia respond well to this injection treatment. The capillaries are effectively removed without any evidence of treatment and usually do not recur.

With more widespread occurrences, which in extreme cases makes the lower limbs look like roadmaps, treatment is more difficult, and the end result not as predictable. In these cases persistence in treatment and patience on the part of the sufferer will yield much improvement. With thorough treatment, even in the most advanced case, 70 to 90% of the blood vessels can often be removed. Patients who want total erradication must return for check-up treatment in order to effect this kind of a result.

The average case, which lies between these two extremes, does well with thorough treatment.

There is a small group who, despite effective treatment and apparent removal of the capillary blemishes, develop a secondary regrowth of blood vessels after a few months which are smaller than the original condition. I have seen some of these cases go on to a tertiary, still finer, vascular regrowth of almost invisible telangiectatic capillaries. This is a rare development affecting only a few individuals who have capillaries that are closely spaced without any isolated branches or clusters. They are more like an angioma at this stage and cannot be treated by the micro-injection technique any further.

Aside from this rare type, telangiectasia responds well to micro-injection therapy.

---

* Phlebographic studies by Ken P. Biegeleisen disclose the presence of feeder arterioles below these blemishes. These must be injected with caution (Personal communication, 1983).

Chapter 14

▪ COSMETIC ASPECTS OF VARICOSE VEINS, CAPILLARIES, AND LYMPH LEG

It is surprising how many women and men have presented themselves for treatment of varicose veins primarily for cosmetic reasons. These individuals often have psychological disturbances which add weight to the importance of their treatment.

Early in my experience attention was drawn to cosmetic problems by the patients themselves. After completing the standard treatment for varicose veins to my satisfaction, the patient often expressed unhappiness over some small venous or capillary enlargements that persisted. I was often entreated to develop a special technique for the management of these smaller vascular disfigurements. To the lay mind, these small surface blemishes were part of the original varicose vein condition.

I found it almost imperative, as far back as 1934, to find a way of dealing with the problem. Micro-injection for telangiectasia was developed, and has withstood the test of time successfully as it is still in use today (Chapter 15).

The recent awareness of the chronicity of varicose veins, plus the fact that surgery is not producing life-long benefits, has made injections acceptable once again. Every visible vein, venule, or capillary can be removed by injection treatment with the proper technique. From a cosmetic viewpoint, sclerotherapy is the most effective method as it leaves no evidence of treatment.

Venules

When it comes to small venules on the lower extremities, injection therapy is also the only practical method to consider. These tiny blood vessels are not usually true varicosities but are dilated, small, superficial veins which have become visible. They usually appear as straight, blue or purple lines with some tortuosity in the larger ones. Because venules add little to the problem of venous insufficiency, they are distinctly a cosmetic problem.

They have been largely neglected in the past. It is natural for many patients to think that they are true varicose veins. Patients often complain of their unsightly appearance. I have made it a practice to eliminate these blood vessels whenever possible for two reasons. First, they may cause bleeding, sometimes of a serious nature, in the ankle area if the overlying, thin skin is broken. Secondly, if enough blood vessels are involved, the area can become the seat of chronic itching dermatitis.

An annoying characteristic of dilated venules is their tendency to come and go depending upon the amount of fluid in the vascular system. Women may find these tiny blood vessels much more conspicuous prior to menstruation when they store fluid. Afterward, the venules are either completely gone or found with great difficulty. This is a problem for the therapist who must sometimes advise the patients to return during the week prior to menstruation.

Treatment of dilated venules is different from that in varicose veins. These blood vessels cannot tolerate strong solutions. The injections must be perfectly made to avoid blistering or sloughing. Sometimes in the delicate skin areas around the ankles, an apparently perfect injection with a strong irritant like sodium morrhuate or Sotradecol will cause blistering or a small area of necrosis. It is necessary to use the weakest agent that will produce sclerosis. I favor solutions like dextrose, 50%; sugar/salt mixtures; diluted fatty acid reagents like 1% sodium morrhuate or 1% Aethoxysklerol.

The needle must be small, from 25 to 30 gauge. The injections are usually made in the upright position, but for the smallest venules approaching capillary size, it may be necessary to lie the patient down and work under magnification.

Successful treatment of dilated venules can be one of the most difficult techniques in sclerotherapy. These blood vessels, especially in the case of neurotic individuals, may well be the bane of the vascular specialist's existence. It is often necessary to wait for an opportunity during the female patient's monthly cycle to locate and inject them. Curiously enough, there are perceptive patients who can find dilated venules when the doctor himself cannot. In my experience, in cases of disagreement, the patient is usually right.

Capillary Enlargements – Telangiectasia

Telangiectasia is an interesting and unsightly capillary condition which has been fully described in the previous chapter (Chapter 13). The end result, if skillfully done, is a normal appearing limb. This may be a major turning point in some women's lives psychologically.

Vascular Blotches

After painstakingly treating varicose veins and telangiectasia of the lower limbs, there are a number of individuals who will still be left with one or more unsightly, reddish or purplish, irregular areas which defy classification. I cannot find a more suitable name than "blotches." They resemble flat angiomata, yet their frequent association with varicose limbs that have dilated venules and capillaries brings them into our vascular realm.

These blotches do not always respond to the treatment to be described. The prognosis depends upon the depth of the involved blood vessels. A rough test of the depth of involvement is to try the effect of finger pressure. If the blotched area can be blanched by simple pressure, then the chance of effective treatment is good. Approximately 50% of these blotched areas can be cured by the following treatment.

Actual blood vessels that can be isolated should be injected directly. A small venule or perhaps a group of capillaries can sometimes be identified in the discolored area or leading to it. They should be treated by appropriate sclerotherapy intravascularly. For the actual blotch or blush, it is necessary to inject subcutaneously and perivascularly for relief. The solution of choice is Aethoxysklerol, from 0.5 to 1% in amounts of 0.5 to 1 c.c. depending upon the size of the area. If the discolored area seems fairly superficial and does not cover more than one-half inch in diameter, the operator should inject approximately 0.5 to 1 c.c. of 1% of this sclerosing solution. In any case, it should produce a whealing reaction to temporarily blanch the lesion. Enough of these wheals are made to cover part or all of the area. This may suffice to clear a mild condition. If not, the treatment is repeated one or more times.

In the deeper seated and more extensive lesions, we have to increase the strength of the sclerosing solution carefully and also increase the amount injected. These two adjustments will depend upon the experience of the operator. The treatment hinges on the ability of most tissues to withstand limited perivascular injection with Aethoxysklerol, 0.5 to 1%.

It will be found following injection that the tissues look congested temporarily. This is controlled by the application of an ice-pack for five minutes. Occasionally it becomes necessary to inject 1% Xylocaine to offset the irritation of the sclerosing solution.

Around the ankle joint it is necessary to exercise even greater care because there is no underlying cushion of subcutaneous fat to protect the blotchy area. All these refinements are a matter of judgment which will tax the skill of the practitioner. Some of the blotches are so deeply placed and are so extensively anastamotic as to defy treatment. It is extremely gratifying when the therapy is successful because after completing sclerotherapy for a varicose limb, any blotches that are present stand out flagrantly to the annoyance of both doctor and patient.

Two other conditions that should be mentioned in discussing cosmetic aspects of this work are lymphedema and unilateral enlargement of the lower limb. These are discussed under their appropriate headings in Chapter 12.

The last complication to be described is pigmentation accompanying lymph leg. While generally considered as irreversible, this has not proven the case in my experience. Depigmentation may sometimes be achieved by appropriate treatment which will be described below.

Depigmentation of Lymphedema

The pigmentation arising in lymph legs is due to the disintegration of red blood cells that are trapped by the pathologic thickening of the subcutaneous tissues in which early forms of fibrosis play a prominent part.

These areas, which may be likened to a low-grade lymphangitis, are relatively soft at first and become more hardened in time as mature connective tissue develops and contracts. Finally, the intractible stage of hard lymphedema appears and the pigmentation is then permanent.

In the early phase of this condition, when the tissues are semi-soft, the injection treatment described in Chapter 12 promotes the absorption of exudates by stimulating the new growth of capillaries and lymphatics, which acts to heal the lesion. It is during this phase before the tissues are densely sclerotic, that the granules of iron (hemosiderin) and other cellular debris are phagocyted and ultimately absorbed from the area. This process gradually removes the brown pigmented appearance from the surface of the lesion. As described previously, the tissues become softer and more normal in appearance. Thus, an area of brown colored limb, which is usually considered an irreversible lesion, can be lightened in color and the tissues reversed to a more normal outward appearance.

With persistent treatment, early areas of lymphedema may be normalized in appearance and color. In many cases of lymph leg, even with moderately advanced pigmentation, the operator will notice a lightening of discoloration accompanying thorough injection treatment. When not restored to a normal appearance, some improvement occurs in most of these legs.

Varicosities of the Hands

Occasionally, women will request treatment for enlarged veins on the back of the hands and wrists for cosmetic reasons. These women complain that this condition, which is popularly associated with old age, makes them look old. There are no symptoms.

While I never suggest treating this condition, in sensitive women it is a factor in creating unhappiness. These are not varicosities, but rather venous enlargements arising as a result of the absorption of subcutaneous fat in the dorsum of the hands. While it is occasionally present in younger women, prominent veins are most often found after the menopause and are associated with aging.

These veins may be successfully sclerosed by the injection of 0.5 to 1 c.c. of sodium morrhuate solution, or a similar amount of 1% Sotradecol. As the veins have a marked tendency to roll aside from the needle point due to the lack of fat under the skin, special measures may be needed to immobilize them. This may consist of tourniquets placed proximally, combined with digital pressure to tighten the skin near the point of injection.

In difficult cases, an assistant may help to hold the skin taut while the operator penetrates the skin first and then using a sharp thrust pierces the vein wall entering its lumen. Gauze sponges strapped down with plastic or elastic adhesive strips are kept in place for three to five days.

The veins that are treated generally respond by sclerosis and absorption for successful effacement.

PART TWO ■ SCLEROTHERAPY

Chapter 15

■ FASCIAL WEAKNESS

Most physicians are familiar with the numerous structural weaknesses to which the human body falls heir. It is becoming increasingly clear that these are not isolated conditions, but have a common etiology and may be grouped into one disease. A group of these conditions associated with connective tissue frailty have been assembled. The term *fascial weakness* (70) appropriately describes this group of diseases and constitutes a new clinical entity.

Varicose veins, hemorrhoids, varicocele, rectocele, cystocele, pes planus, low back syndrome, various ptoses, herniae and scoliosis of the spine are among the numerous evidences of this inherited stromal deficiency. Persons with one of these disorders have a relatively high incidence of one or more of the others. They are all characterized by a failure of the supporting fascia to resist environmental forces. This disrupts the integrity of the affected organs and the body in general.

These environmental forces are an additional strain on the connective tissue supporting structure of the body. Man, in his evolutionary climb to the upright posture, has never fully adapted himself to these additional strains. Since the natural selective forces of evolution do not play a dominant role in man's civilized environment, the result has been that individuals with inadequacies of the supporting tissues have not been eliminated but have survived. Support for this viewpoint is found in the fact that the many and various evidences of fascial weakness found in man do not present themselves in the lower animal forms. For example, according to veterinarians and zookeepers, varicose veins are practically unknown in animals.

CONNECTIVE TISSUE

The study of connective tissue has shed new light on fascial weakness. This field now deserves and requires the attention it has long been denied. Ligaments and tendons have virtually been dismissed as "lifeless" because, like the long bones, they are largely proteinaceous fibers in amorphous ground substance with relatively few interspersed cells. However the situation has changed and many workers are now concentrating their efforts on the connective tissue system, which has been recognized as a dynamic one. It is now considered quite alive and susceptible to pathological disorders.

The most characteristic elements in connective tissue are the fibers. The three varieties are: collagenous, elastic and reticular. The function of the first, or collagenous type, is to provide rigid support. As the name implies, elastic fibers provide resilience as well as support in areas which require an ability to adjust to local strains and stresses. The third type, reticular fibers, form a separating layer between connective and adjacent tissue.

Collagen

The structure of collagen, on the molecular level, has now been elucidated as a complex protein macromolecule. It forms the tropocollagen molecule consisting of three left-handed helices wound together as a right-handed superhelix (71). The collagen fibrils are formed of these basic building blocks. They possess considerable elasticity in themselves but form larger fibers which rigidly resist stretching when they aggregate normally. Thus, being composed largely of collagen, most ligaments of the body will tear before they stretch appreciably.

We have known for years that, embryonically, connective tissue arises from mesenchyme cells. These are cells of irregular form and wandering habits which originate in the mesodermal somites and lateral plates of the embryo. The three primary tissue layers are the first residence of the mesenchyme cells. Even at this early phase, a wandering tendency is displayed by these cells which give rise to collagenous tissue.

Fibroblasts, in the mature individual, are also cells of a wandering nature and are the sites of synthesis of tropocollagen molecules. They then form collagen fibrils by aggregating extracellularly. Fibroblasts, which enter into scar tissue formation throughout the body, give considerable evidence of rising from nucleated blood cells. Observed in cultures of the buffy coat layer from centrifuged blood specimens are transitional forms from lymphocytes and monocytes to fibroblasts and, eventually, sheets of connective tissue. The inhibition of scar formation further evidences this transition in experimental wounds in animals subjected to total body irradiation which destroys nucleated blood cells.

Reticulin and Elastin

The characteristic component of reticular fibers, reticulin, has not been as widely considered as collagen. An immaturity has been implied by the fact that reticular fibers are frequently found in the sites of accumulation of undifferentiated cells of mesenchymal nature. Some have even suggested that these are "precollagenous" fibers.

The predominant tissue in such organs as the aorta is elastic tissue which has as its characteristic component the albumoid elastin. Like collagen, elastin may develop from a precursor secreted by the fibroblasts. (73) These tissues elastin and collagen, are thought by some workers to be different developmental stages of the same basic form. Future research should determine the exact nature of elastin.

Hormones in Fascial Weakness

Previous experience with the treatment of varicose veins stimulated our present inquiry into fascial weakness. Many years of observation have shown me that an inherited weakness of the fascial supporting tissue of the vein walls is a basic defect in varicose veins. Other workers in the field have made similar findings.

Some investigators reporting in the literature theorize that hormonal factors play an important role in causing varicose veins and other fascial defects. The influence of these factors on varicose veins is seen in the different sexes by the rapid appearance of varicose veins in pregnancy and in the intensification of the varicose veins condition during menstruation.

The first study of the composition of varicose vein walls was probably done by Svejcar and his associates. (74) Their interesting results showed that, when compared by percentage composition to normals, varicose vein walls have a deficiency in collagen content. Furthermore, they found that unaffected veins from persons with varices elsewhere on the body also showed this deficiency but not as markedly as in the actual varix wall.

The Svejcar study strongly suggests that varicose veins might be caused by a collagen deficiency since collagen is assumed to provide structural support for blood vessels and because varicose veins are characterized by distention to the point where valve leaflets no longer meet effectively. The summary of his significant findings is as follows:

1) Decreased concentration of collagen.
2) Increased concentration of water.
3) Increased hexosamine content.

An interesting note is that the symptomatic dilatation of varicose veins seems also to be a characteristic response of the uterine cervix to pregnancy, at which time varicosities often also make an appearance. Strikingly similar to the above described investigation of varicose veins are the results of several metabolic studies of the cervices of gravid rats. The following changes were noted, in addition to increased dilatability and decrease in tensile strength:

1) Decreased concentration of collagen.
2) Increased concentration of water.
3) Relative increase in hexosamine content.

Similar changes have been brought about in the cervices of non-gravid rats by treatment with the hormone relaxin, following estrogen priming. The addition of progesterone to the therapy causes the values to approach those seen in actual pregnancy.

The rather startling similarity of the changes in the gravid cervix to the changes in varicose veins mentioned above suggests a hormonal influence in the evolution of this disease. This factor seems to be associated with pregnancy, and we would therefore expect, if our reasoning is correct, that other fascial structures should be affected at the same time. That this is the case is indicated by the following findings during pregnancy, related to the connective tissue structures:

1) Decrease in the tensile strength of the cervix, and other changes mentioned above.

2) Decrease in tensile strength of the skin.

3) Striking increase in the incidence of dissecting aortic aneurysm. (Among women, half of these occur during pregnancy).

4) Similar increase in incidence of ruptured splenic artery aneurysm.

5) Frequent appearance of varicose veins.

6) Frequent onset of backache.

7) Relaxation of the ligaments of the symphysis pubis.

As noted, the relaxation of the symphyeal ligaments, resulting in pubic separation is caused by the production of relaxin. (75) In fact, it was the study of pubic separation which led to the discovery of relaxin. This hormone seems to have a general loosening effect on those areas connected with childbirth. There is also evidence that the sacroiliac ligaments are affected. Complaints of lower back pain were observed by Chamberlain (76) to accompany pubic separation, especially before menstruation.

Relaxin causes a cleavage and dissolution of the collagen fibres. (77) Its tendency to loosen connective tissue, its apparent connection with backache, and its appearance during menstruation and pregnancy suggest that this hormone may well be a factor in the production of fascial weakness. Other hormones have also been shown to affect the fascia. We will understand fascial disorders much better if we learn more about these various hormonal interactions.

The pituitary and adrenal hormones provide a few examples of this. Deoxycorticosterone acetate stimulates proliferation and activity of fibroblasts in connective tissue repair. (78) Cortisone, on the other hand, exerts effects which seem to be antagonistic. It inhibits fibroblast proliferation and production of collagen.

Somatotropin, a pituitary hormone, causes changes opposing cortisone, and corticotropin seems to oppose these changes. Our understanding of hormonal effect on fascia is quite incomplete. This is therefore a fruitful area for future research on this problem.

Collagen Diseases

Because of their similarity to the group of diseases we have been discussing mention should be made of the collagen group. Here, the hereditary factor is even more pronounced, or at least more apparent, than in fascial weakness, perhaps because of the severity of the symptoms.

Marfan's syndrome, characterized by dissecting aortic aneurysm, herniae, scoliosis, and other fascial defects, is an example. Severe varicose veins may also be present. (79)

Supporting the thesis that varicose veins, flat feet, herniae, and other diseases mentioned at the beginning of this discussion are related disorders, is the coincident occurrence of all these symptoms in so many patients.

The failure of the collagen fibrils to aggregate properly is thought to be the origin of some collagen diseases and hormones have, here also, been suggested as probable causative agents.

The treatment of fascial disorders by injection has caused more confusion and dissension than in any other field of therapy. Sclerotherapy which is now practiced throughout the world has undergone a modification in recent years which is termed *prolotherapy*. In this altered concept new tissue results from the usual irritants used in sclerotherapy, which are replaced by weaker chemical irritants. This is supposed to stimulate the proliferation of new tendo-osseous tissue which repairs and strengthens the weakened areas.

The result has been that there are now two schools of thought in sclerosing procedures. Sclerotherapy is the acceptable term for the treatment of varicose veins and capillary disorders, while injection treatment for other diseases elsewhere in the body is now discussed under two headings. There is no dispute over the degree of chemical irritation for most soft tissue conditions like bursitis with effusion, and fissure or ganglion, but differences of opinion have arisen for the treatment of tendon and fascial repair.

Basically the opposing camps are divided over the strength of chemical irritation, even though the same sclerosing agent may be used by both. Based upon animal experiments which I began in 1956 (80), using fatty-acid solutions like Sylnasol in rabbit tendons, I reported the growth of new tendon tissue within two months of treatment. Borden (81) subsequently confirmed this finding which supports the cause of prolotherapy adherents.

I favor more potent solutions like zinc-phenol mixtures for tendons and aim at new tissue in addition to fibrosis. It will be difficult to reach a conclusion because more study is needed which will take considerable time.

Types of Tissue Repair

Not enough attention has been paid to the different types of scar tissue that the human body is capable of forming in the healing process. There are at least seven kinds of tissue repair, and probably more, deserving intensive future study. Some of these are properly discussed here in the context of sclerotherapy. Others are beyond the scope of this book but are included to make the group complete.

They can be listed as follows:

1) Scar following surgery.
2) Excessive scar in keloid formation.
3) Scar following sclerotherapy.
4) Tissue repair following prolotherapy.
5) Epithelial scar following trauma in infancy and childhood.
6) Skin scar resulting from injury in adult.
7) Tissue repair by regeneration.

As noted above the difference between prolotherapy and sclerotherapy resides in the promotion of tissue growth in one (prolotherapy) and the development of scar tissue in the other (sclerotherapy).

It is my thought that it is not possible to secure one without the other to some degree. Thus, if the injection stimulates the growth of new tendon tissue, there will be an attendant connective tissue response as well, in the form of some degree of scarring.

The controversy between the supporters of mild sclerosing therapy versus those who favor stronger chemicals is in an early phase and will be resolved only with continued study as noted above.

There is obviously a hormonal influence at play in the repair process of the human body. For example, I have noticed white, thick scars on the legs of patients who gave a history of having received the original injury during childhood. The same kind of trauma in adult life often heals with minimal or no scarring. This is such a characteristic finding that the discerning physician can pick out childhood scars on simple examination. There is no other explanation than different hormonal response to account for this. The scars of childhood are obviously different than those produced in later life. Yet, following surgery, dense scarring takes place over the incisions in young and old. A different healing process has been initiated by incising the tissues. The tissue juices resulting from interruption of the continuity of the skin, subcutaneous tissue, fascial layers, muscles, together with blood vessels, nerves and lymphatics release other hormones which stimulate the densest type of scar tissue.

The nature of the hormone and healing response to incisional injury is different from relatively minor superficial tissue damage, and the scar tissue reaction varies correspondingly. We do not fully understand tissue repair, but it seems to be controlled by hormones which are released upon cellular division or necrosis.

It is obvious that chemical irritation is not the ideal way to secure proliferating or scar tissue. It is my feeling that continued research in this area will point the way to the development of direct hormonal stimulation of new tissue or scar tissue as the case may be. It is important to note that steroids retard scar tissue formation, which in fact may be an entering wedge in the direction of improvement of sclerosing solutions. The study of cortisone antagonists like deoxycorticosterone could well lead to further developments in this field.

Other examples of tissue repair by non-chemical methods will be discussed in the future of sclerotherapy (Chapter 27).

The solutions that I and others have developed, and the techniques associated with them, are nevertheless quite successful in achieving their goals, at the present time. Future improvement by hormonal stimulation of the body's repair processes will improve this picture further.

Chapter 16

▪ HEMORRHOIDS AND RECTAL PROLAPSE

Sclerotherapy for hemorrhoids is a well-known procedure to most doctors. General practitioners as well as proctologists have given wide acceptance to the sclerosing method of treatment.

There is some difficulty in judging the percentage of hemorrhoidal cases receiving the injection form of treatment at this time. Nevertheless, one can estimate that between 50 and 75% are being treated by this method using existing techniques with, occasionally, some minor office surgery added. The addition of my improved technique that ensures greater success will encourage wider use of this therapy in office practice.

Some thirty years ago, the injection method for treatment of hemorrhoids was partly in the hands of "quacks" and "irregulars." With the introduction of safer sclerosing agents, medical acceptance has become widespread.

As I have pointed out previously (82), internal hemorrhoids, like other varicosities, have their etiology in inherited fascial weakness. This correlation is often evidenced in the family history, which may show parents suffering from varicose veins and other fascial disorders.

Depending on the physician's point of view, other causes are frequently mentioned. Pregnancy may be deemed responsible for the development of hemorrhoids in the viewpoint of the obstetrician. The importance of constipation or diarrhea may be emphasized by the gastroenterologist. The increase in venous pressure in the hemorrhoidal vessels may be attributed to man's upright posture. Other etiological factors that are mentioned are venous obstruction as in liver cirrhosis or infection as in cryptitis.

The average practitioner has no difficulty in recognizing a case of hemorrhoids. Pain and bleeding are the most frequent symptoms exhibited. Thromboses of external piles are a frequent cause of pain. Bleeding from upper bowel lesions must be carefully separated from that of hemorrhoidal bleeding. A bright red color is an important diagnostic sign of rectal bleeding, but a more positive finding would be locating the bleeding vessel by speculum examination. Without such visualization, the physician can only assume that the bleeding is hemorrhoidal in origin when it cannot be traced to any other source.

Where prolapse has occurred and internal piles, covered by a mucous membrane, have protruded from the anus in a mass, simple inspection of the anal region will often make the diagnosis. Digital examination using a wide sweeping motion will reveal the soft, boggy mass of internal hemorrhoids, conveying a characteristic sensation. Using one of a variety of rectal speculae, diagnosis can usually be confirmed by anoscopic examination. I usually prefer the Brinkerhoff speculum which, because of its convenient slide opening, is also useful for treatment.

Hemorrhoids are readily discerned under anoscopic examination as bulging, well-rounded, venous masses within the anorectal canal, having various configurations. Occasionally, blue-walled, bulging varices may be readily recognized as veins. At other times, glistening, white or pink, compressible bulges may be seen. During examination, various degrees of prolapse may be noted. Where marked stretching of the rectal lining has occurred, the hemorrhoidal masses may be displaced for a considerable distance with the motion of the speculum as the operator advances or withdraws the instrument.

The anal canal, the terminal portion of the large intestine, lies below the rectum, with an oval aperture which is called the anus. Up to the anorectal line, the anal canal is lined by both true and modified skin. The internal sphincter closes one end of the canal and the external sphincter, with its familiar outside corrugations, the other end.

The support of the anal canal is the levator ani muscle. The white line of Hilton is the juncture where the internal sphincter overlaps the external sphincter. It appears at the junction of the middle with the lower third of the anal canal. The whole area curves backward and is 3 cm. long. This curvature is the cause of the difficulty in injecting internal hemorrhoids through a rectal speculum.

The anal canal is surrounded by the external and internal sphincter muscles. The canal is in relation to the levator ani muscles and the anal coccygeal gland, posteriorly. The canal is separated, laterally, from the ischiorectal fossae by the anal fascia. The urethral bulb, the urogenital diaphragm, the prostatic apex, the anterior fibers of the levator ani, and the perineal body are found anteriorly in the male. In the female, the fibromuscular perineal body separates the lower end of the canal from the vagina, anteriorly. The sphincter muscles are present in every direction because they encircle the anal canal.

There are, in general, three types of internal hemorrhoids; the vascular type having a red raspberry appearance in which vascular tissue predominates; the polypoid type in which the tumors are pedunculated, the top being larger than the base; and the mixed type.

Internal hemorrhoids are, generally, varicosities of one or more radicles of the superior hemorrhoidal veins. They arise above the anorectal line and are covered by mucous membrane. In some cases, however, they may develop from the middle and inferior hemorrhoidal plexuses and are found lower down in the canal.

The connection between the sigmoid and the anal canal is the rectum. The rectal wall has four layers: peritoneal, muscular, submucosal, and mucosal. Its origin is opposite the third sacral vertebra and it curves down around the concavity of the sacrum and coccyx joining the anal canal at the anorectal line. When stretched out at autopsy, it measures 6 inches (15 cm.). In the live specimen, the average is 5.4 inches due to the curvature present. At the rectosigmoid junction it expands, being at its smallest above that. At its lowest point, the juncture with the anal canal, it once again narrows. The chief support for the rectum and the anus is the levator ani muscle and the external sphincter.

Posteriorly, the rectum is in relation with the hemorrhoidal vessels, pyriformis muscle, sacral nerves, sacrum coccyx, and levator ani. Anteriorly, in the male, it is adjacent to the bladder, triangular ligament, prostate and the seminal vesicles. In the female, anteriorly, it is in relation with the small intestine, uterus, vagina, and, laterally, with the ureters, internal iliac artery and branches, obturator internus muscle and nerve.

The rectum presents two curves laterally; the upper sacral and the lower perineal. The upper is concave anteriorly and the lower is concave posteriorly. Viewed from the anterior aspect, there are three lateral curves, two on the left and a third, in the middle, on the right.

The anatomical factors outlined above are not taken into consideration in current methods of injection therapy for internal hemorrhoids and prolapse. The curvatures of the anorectal tube produce a limiting effect on angles of injection which is not appreciated. Not fully understood either, is the importance of the neighboring structures in relation to the origin and correction of these defects. This is the case, particularly, in rectal prolapse which presents a special difficulty in effective sclerosing therapy.

Abnormal descent of the rectal mucosa through the anus is termed prolapse. The descent of the rectum with all its coats through the anal orifice is termed procidentia. In either of these events, there may or may not be protrusion. The number of coats of the bowel involved therefore, makes the distinction. Prolapse is downward mucosal sliding; procidentia is a slipping of the whole wall. Anywhere from the modified skin of the anal canal to the rectum or sigmoid may be the area of involvement. An actual intusseption or invagination may occur if the condition is extensive or high enough. Children more often develop prolapse and adults, procidentia.

A condition of prolapse may develop into one of procidentia. In the latter, the defect is in the fascial, muscular, or peritoneal supports of the bowel. Prolapse develops in children due to the loose fixation of the peri-rectal tissues and the vertical course of the rectum. An extensive procidentia in adults is analogous to a sliding hernia.

Internal prolapse, which feels like a double layer of mucosa to the examiner, does not protrude. In spite of the reduplication or looseness of the mucous membrane, the wall of the anus or rectum is palpated as intact. A protruding prolapse is considered an external prolapse and is noticed on defecation. It remains out rather constantly in advanced cases, unless it is reposited manually. It may not be possible to reposit the prolapse in extreme cases, the parts having become thickened and histologically changed.

To diagnose a procidentia which protrudes, one may look for a series of circular folds and a mass larger and more extensive than that in a prolapse. To detect an internal procidentia, a digital examination is conducted in a squatting or sitting position. The involvement of the entire rectal wall can then be felt in the mass. In addition, the extrusion is thicker, firmer, and movable.

Technique

The usual technique for the injection treatment of hemorrhoids is as follows: Insert into the anal canal a well-lubricated speculum of the operator's choice. The Martin or Brinkerhoff types are the most popular in average use today. On exposing the hemorrhoidal tissue, the needle is inserted into the upper portion of the hemorrhoidal mass for about 1/8 to 1/4 inch. This is considered by most authors as a submucosal injection. This is the average technique, with some variations, that is universally in use for injection therapy of internal hemorrhoids.

This method deals most effectively with simple hemorrhoidal masses. Where the condition is advanced or where rectal prolapse has occurred, it may fail. The medical profession has accepted these facts, with complacency, for many years and has actually judged prolapse to be a contraindication to injection treatment. The reasons for failing were never fully appreciated.

It was physically impossible to perform the deeper injections required with this standard technique. In cases of rectal prolapse, the older technique failed more often than it cured.

Older therapists, oddly enough, were cognizant of the fact that deeper injections were needed in children for the treatment of rectal prolapse. In 1928, Hanes (83) suggested using a solution of 1:3000 hydrochloric acid for injection of the perirectal structures on both sides of the rectum. In 1932, Gabriel (84) also suggested perirectal injection but used a quinine-sulfuric acid solution. In 1933, Potter (85), working under anesthesia, inserted a long needle through the perianal skin about 1/2 inch lateral to the anal margin for a depth of about 2 or 3 inches. Modern therapists accepted the limitations of the current injection methods without question and, surprisingly, never appreciated the significance and value of deep injection therapy for their adult patients.

Anatomically we have seen that the anal and rectal canals are built upon a series of curves. Extrinsic structures, which include fascial and muscular tissue, provide support for the walls of these canals. A bed is formed by the submucous coat of the rectum, upon which the mucosa rests and, with its loose attachment, allows the mucosa to slide. Therefore, it becomes important to inject deeply enough to reach the supporting structures of these canals. This is not possible with currently accepted injection methods.

A barrier to the deep penetration of anorectal tissue is the series of curves which is the target area for injection. In addition, the bulge of tissue that protrudes into the mouth of the rectal speculum consists, usually, of mucosa only, with or without submucosa. This mass is connected only in a loose fashion with the underlying structures and is movable and difficult to transfix. It is not uncommon for the therapist to pierce through the hemorrhoid completely as he attempts to inject the structure.

The confining area of the rectal speculum itself is the source of the worst drawback of current injection therapy. The Brinkerhoff speculum shows this clearly. When one uses a 3 c.c. syringe and a hemorrhoidal needle, the needle lies in a cone-shaped space narrower at the pointed end of the speculum. The area in which a therapist must work may be from 3/4 to 1 inch in diameter varying with the size of the instrument. The area narrows to about 1/2 inch at the point in the slide in which most injections are made.

Using the floor of the speculum as a longitudinal axis, one will note that the angle of injection which the needle makes will average about 15 degrees. This angle of injection can be increased to about 20 degrees by pulling back the slide of the speculum, thus exposing a greater slot. Upon study of Figure 23, it can be observed that a needle which penetrates a pile at the

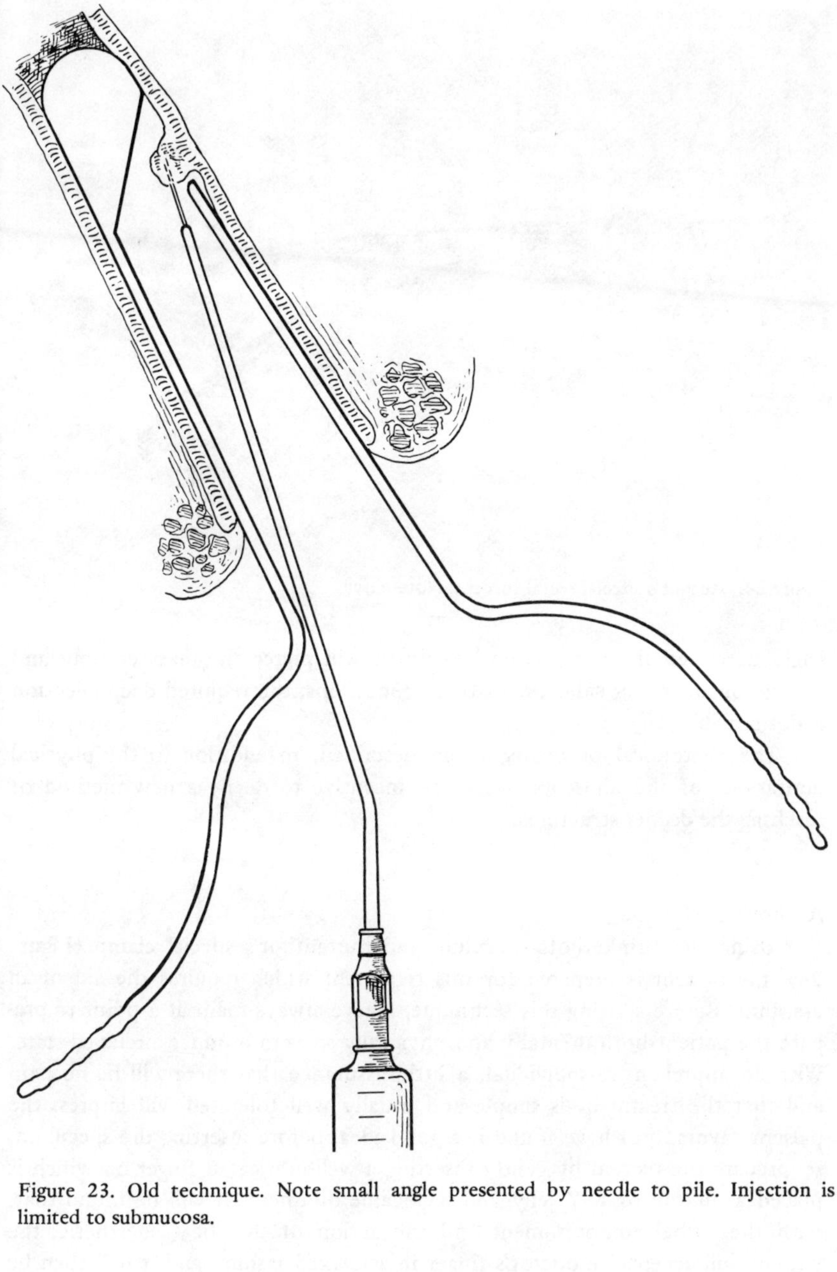

Figure 23. Old technique. Note small angle presented by needle to pile. Injection is limited to submucosa.

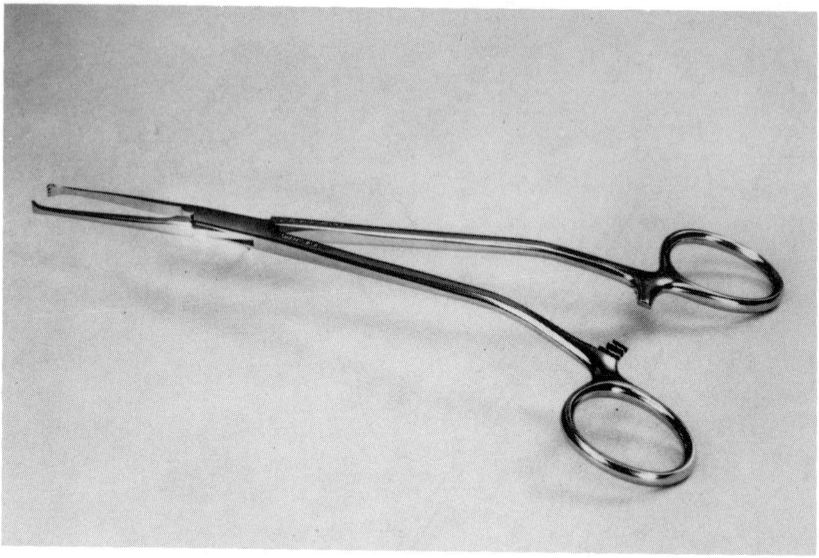

Figure 24. Author's special rectal forceps. Note curve.

angle described is placed submucosally or will pierce the mass entirely and emerge on the other side. Under these conditions, the required deep injection is not possible.

The anatomical problems herein described, in addition to the physical limitations of the anoscope were the incentive to devise a new method of reaching the deeper structures.

Author's Technique

Using the Brinkerhoff speculum and the author's special clamp (Figure 24), the patient is prepared for this treatment which requires the aid of an assistant. Before starting this technique, I have always made it a point to prepare the patient both mentally and physically so as to produce a relaxed state. With an apprehensive individual, a little assurance that there will be no pain and that the treatment is simple and usually well tolerated will impress the patient favorably. I have found it a good idea, before inserting the speculum, to prepare the rectum by gently inserting a well-lubricated finger on which is placed a mixtue of K-Y jelly and Xylocaine ointment. It will be found that, with the verbal admonishment and the action of the local anesthetic, the patient will accept the doctor's finger in a relaxed fashion and it will then be possible to dilate the orifice so there will be no pain upon the introduction of the speculum. The patient himself will indicate his readiness for the treatment by breathing comfortably and offering a relaxed anal sphincter.

At this point the Brinkerhoff speculum is gently inserted, either to its full length in one motion, or in degrees if there is still some slight resistance.

Checking that the floor lamp is properly focused, with the light coming over the doctor's right shoulder if he is right-handed, and the assistant conveniently placed alongside the operator, the slide of the speculum is opened to expose the area of treatment with its protruding hemorrhoid within the slot. The hemorrhoid is now grasped with the special Allis-type clamp which I have devised for this technique.

The handle of this clamp is bent away from the speculum to allow room for the introduction of a long hemorrhoid needle alongside it for the actual injection. Since one is working in the confines of a narrow canal with two instruments in place having different functions and different motions, it became necessary to bend the handle for proper viewing of the procedure. It is therefore important to have an assistant previously trained for this special technique who will hold the clamp in place while the doctor makes the injection (Figure 25).

The actual procedure is as follows: The operator will grasp the pile with the altered Allis clamp (Biegeleisen clamp). He then hands it to his assistant who brings the hemorrhoid, with its submucosal base, into view within the slot of the speculum by a special motion. Ordinary traction will not do this at all. It is necessary to press the handle and its adjoining blades against the side of the speculum, pushing paradoxically in the opposite direction to where the pile will present itself. The bottom of the instrument wall becomes a fulcrum which will aid in swinging the tip of the clamp toward the center of the slot, bringing the pile into view for injection.

The operator is now holding the speculum with one hand while he makes the injection with the other. The combined maneuver, which requires three hands, cannot be performed by a doctor working alone.

I have used many sclerosing solutions for this injection treatment and found that phenolized oil is the most efficient and safe one for this therapy. Other workers employ Sotrodecol, 1 to 3%, or Quinine-Urea-Hydrochloride, 5%. I sometimes resort to these two solutions myself in the event of allergy or sensitivity to the phenol solution. Any of the standard fatty acid solutions that are used for varicose veins are also suitable for careful injection treatment of hemorrhoids. The oil bases for the phenol solution may be olive oil, almond oil, or cottonseed oil. I prefer almond or cottonseed oil.

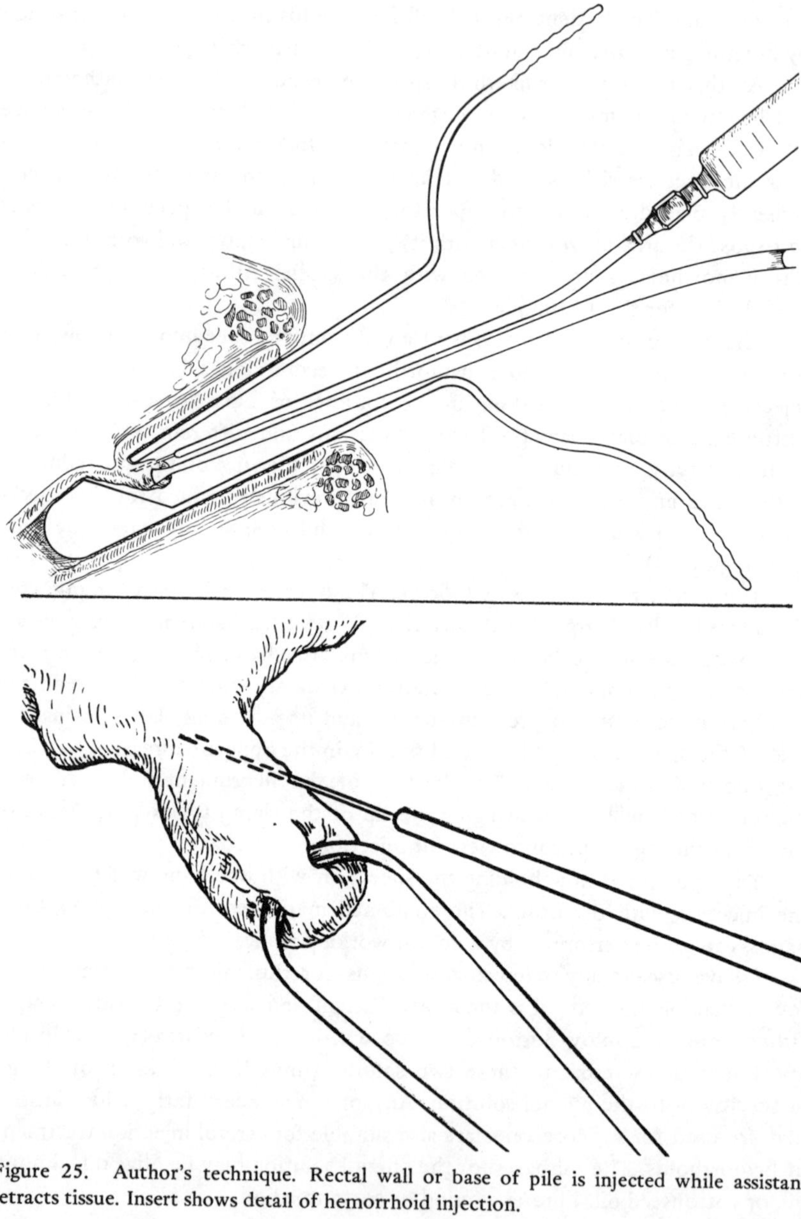

Figure 25. Author's technique. Rectal wall or base of pile is injected while assistant retracts tissue. Insert shows detail of hemorrhoid injection.

The amount injected will vary from 0.5 to 2 c.c. of phenol, 5 to 8%, in cottonseed oil. Other oil bases are not desirable since they may produce oleomas.

When the injection is finished, the clamp is first released, after which the needle and speculum are withdrawn. This procedure may be repeated two or three times during a session. Sometimes the same pile or prolapsed pile may have to be re-injected a few times before sufficient sclerosing is established to shrink it completely. The size of the speculum selected will vary with the degree of involvement. Longer instruments will be needed for piles arising higher up in the canal and appropriate smaller sizes for smaller or younger individuals.

There is a similarity between this technique and surgery. In surgery, usually, the hemorrhoid is grasped and held taut while the base of the mass is treated in a variety of ways. Likewise, in the technique I advocate, the base is similarly exposed and treated rather than just the upper tip of the hemorrhoid which is usually presented by the speculum. This was not achieved by earlier injection methods.

Weekly injections are administered using this clamp method of treatment. There will be little or no reaction to the treatment as the dexterity of the therapist increases. In my experience, most patients are comfortable with this treatment given once a week. This may be increased to twice weekly for the simple method of injection treatment without the clamp or ordinary submucosal injections can be alternated with the deeper clamp method. Sloughing has been rare in my experience. It may be prevented by carefully selecting the area to be treated and the amount injected. Where it occurs, healing is usually prompt and is aided by the submucosal infiltration of 1% Procaine solution. The important point, is not to inject near the surface of the mucosa, but to aim for the deeper layers.

The clamp technique will reduce the number of treatments required for a case of hemorrhoids. Where previously a moderately advanced case of hemorrhoids required 10 to 15 injections, this approach will reduce it to perhaps 6 injections.

Rectal Prolapse

As described previously, abnormal descent of the rectal mucosa through the anus is termed prolapse. This is in contrast to the dropping of the rectum with all its coats when it is termed procidentia. The distinction is therefore made by the number of layers of the bowel wall that are involved. Another way to look at it is that prolapse is a sliding of the inner lining of the canal rather than a slipping of the entire wall.

It is not necessary for the prolapsed mucosa to protrude through the anus for it to be troublesome to the patient. As a rule, he is not aware of the condition unless it happens during defecation. If the condition is not relieved, it has a tendency to advance until the prolapsed mucosa remains outside permanently even though the patient pushes it in after bowel movements.

The technique which I developed was practiced years ago in a modified form (86), but the solutions and technique were different. The technique which I advocate was developed independently and was not inspired by the older methods which were used in children only.

After the patient is positioned in the lateral-prone position, the rectum is prepared in the usual fashion by inserting a lubricated finger on the gloved hand. It is advisable to use the K-Y rectocaine blend mentioned previously. The operator must avoid getting the perianal skin too greasy as this will impede the injections that follow. The anal sphincter is dilated by gently inserting the examining finger and moving it from side to side until no resistance is felt.

With spasm in a nervous patient, it may not be possible to relax the sphincter in this fashion. It then becomes necessary to anesthetize the sphincter by injecting into it 1 or 2% Procaine or Xylocaine solution. This is performed on the mucosal side of the sphincter by injecting a few minims at a time into the four quadrants of the anal canal while traversing in a circular fashion. It may only be necessary to make three or four injections to produce noticeable relaxation.

Having previously identified the area of prolapse which may be present in part of the canal or its entire circumference, the operator starts the procedure by anesthetizing the skin around the anus. For the patient's comfort, I find it advisable to perform this initial anesthesia using a 30 guage needle on a 2 c.c. syringe. This tiny needle should reduce the sensation experienced by the patient to little more than a pin prick. In fact, it is usually well tolerated and, sometimes, not painful at all. I concentrate the anesthesia in the area where the actual perirectal injection will be made. This is done by raising a skin wheal in two or more selected points and, using the wheal as a base, several minims at a time of the usual Xylocaine solution are injected intracutaneously and partially subcutaneously by changing the angle of the needle to cover a small circle around the wheal.

The operator must decide in this perirectal technique how many deep injections will be required to fix the sliding mucosa in the area of prolapse. In mild cases, I usually treat two areas opposite each other. For instance, if about half of the rectal lining slides down toward the anus, let us say on the dorsal aspect, I prefer two injections opposing each other in their horizontal planes so that the points of adhesion will be concentrated at the lateral end of the mucosal looseness. To reinforce this procedure where the laxity of the mucosa covers half of the rectal lining, I sometimes, cautiously, add a third injection if this prolapse involves the dorsal half of the rectum. Obviously, the ventral half which overlies the prostate and bladder is a dangerous area for perirectal injection. It should be avoided. In most cases, reliance must be based upon the lateral sectors of the rectal wall and, even there, extreme care must be observed to travel submucosally and not too deeply.

If the operator is right-handed, he must train his left hand for palpation during this bimanual technique. First, the rectal finger is inserted deeply to palpate the area of mucosa which will be treated. Notice must be taken of its curves and the condition of the wall. Having satisfied himself where he will direct the neddle point, and using a 5 c.c. syringe with a 4 inch, 20 gauge needle containing 1% Xylocaine, the operator pierces the skin previously anesthetized and advances the needle with the external hand in such a fashion that he can feel its presence accurately with the index finger of the gloved hand within the rectum.

The injection of Xylocaine is made while the needle is moving upward, infusing a few minims in a more or less continuous fashion as the advance motion is made. This will not be without pauses. After having covered about 3/4 of an inch, the operator should pause to make certain that the needle point is directly beneath the mucosa and not penetrating it or going away from it too deeply. With practice, and some manual dexterity, the operator will find that he can advance the needle for about 3 inches successfully. This should cause little or no pain because the anesthesia precedes or goes along with the injection.

At this point, the syringe is removed from the inserted needle and another syringe, containing 3 c.c. of sclerosing solution is attached to the hub, and it is now a relatively simple act to withdraw the needle smoothly while at the same time sclerosing solution is continuously injected along its track. Having safely placed the needle during the first half of this procedure one may feel assured that the sclerosing fluid will be deposited into the proper tissues because one is not injecting but withdrawing. The amount of fluid and its sclerosing will vary somewhat depending upon the severity of the prolapse. I have injected 1 to 3 c.c. of phenolized oil of 6 to 8% concentration for 3 inches of injection. This has always been well tolerated.

For the opposite side of the canal, in cases where two injections are deemed necessary, the operator must now reverse his hands so that if he is is right-handed and if the treatment is on the left side of the patient's rectum, the internal guiding finger must be by the right hand while the hand holding the syringe becomes the left hand. The procedure is repeated exactly as before with the hands in reverse and approximately the same amount of fluid is injected. This will suffice for an average, mild case of rectal prolapse. The treatment may be repeated in two weeks and adjustments in amount and strength of the phenol component can be made. Furthermore, if more sclerosing action is desired, the injections can be made closer to each other or even increased in number to a total of three for each half of the canal wall. This does not apply to the lower or ventral half of the rectal canal where one is working in proximity to the bladder and prostate.

It is apparent that for this kind of sclerotherapy, the physician must train his hands bimanually so that either one can make injections. This is also the case for hernial injections (see Chapter 24) where bimanual dexterity is mandatory for anyone attempting the technique.

This sclerosing method is applicable only to mucosal laxity within the reach of the injecting needle. It will have no influence upon rectal prolapse or procidentia higher up in the canal. Therefore, in discussing the prognosis with patients, one must be careful to explain this. On the other hand, individuals with prolapsed mucosa may obtain considerable relief with this method even if the condition arises higher up because it will tack down the lower half or preponderance of loose mucosa thereby holding back the greater part of the prolapse. If the patient will accept this kind of relief, which may be temporary, it can be attempted.

The results of injection treatments for uncomplicated internal hemorrhoids are universally accepted as satisfactory. This method has materially reduced the number of surgical procedures. For the cases of hemorrhoids with prolapse, a combination of injections for internal hemorrhoids combined with the perirectal technique may produce gratifying relief.

Chapter 17

■ FISSURE IN ANO

While an anal fissure appears to be a crack in the anal skin, it is often an ulcer of the entire skin thickness, and is usually found in the posterior anal wall. The crack often lies in the long axis of the anal canal.

Actually there is often an elongated or slit-like split present in the lining of the canal, at and below the anorectal line. It may be found on the front wall of the anus, especially in women, but is least commonly seen in the side walls.

The underlying cause of anal fissure is anal infection which occurs in stages. First, infectious material from the bowel content invades the anal crypts and the tiny ducts and glands attached to them. Following this the infection is carried into the perianal and perirectal tissues by way of the lymphatics or directly through breaks in this area, probably from over distention. Once the infectious material has gained entrance to anal tissues it can localize in the subcutaneous area which may result in destruction of the overlying skin to cause an anal ulcer.

Another mechanism for the development of anal ulcer follows trauma. The thin wall of the crypt tears following the passage of a hard stool.

In the acute stage, the tear in the anal skin may extend through the subcutaneous tissue into the sphincter muscle. The edges are clean, soft and sharply defined; the base is shallow and elastic. At the lower edge of the tear there is often a tag of edematous skin called the *sentinel pile*.

Unless proper treatment is instituted, the fissure fails to heal because of the contracted external sphincter muscle. In the next phase, daily infection and irritation from feces makes the ulcerative tissue thicker and the adjacent anal skin congested. If this painful condition is neglected further a heavy scar tissue develops underneath the ulcer. Scarring makes it difficult for the patient to pass a bowel movement without further tearing. A vicious cycle follows with more tearing, widening and deepening of the ulceration. It is thus important to intervene as soon as possible to prevent this more serious problem.

Pain

Cases of anal ulcer or fissure are not uncommon and because of the pain, are usually seen by the physician in the early stages. This is a fortunate occurrence because treatment can be given promptly.

This characteristic pain, burning in character, is recurrent, often severe, and may last from a few minutes to a few hours. It is usually initiated by defecation and is due to a spasm of the anal sphincter muscles, which continues until they are fatigued and the anus relaxes.

Sometimes a special freedom from pain interval, occurs after defecation if the sphincter muscle does not go into spasm immediately. There is then a gratifying pause up to 1/2 hour when inevitably, it ends with a sudden contraction of the anal sphincter. The cycle of rectal pain returns with extreme incapacitating distress and persists for a variable period up to 2 hours. There may be no further pain until the next bowel movement when the whole picture is repeated.

This pain must be distinguished from that occurring in rectal abscess, and external hemorrhoidal clots. Gross rectal examination will usually identify them.

Anal fissures are usually single. When multiple, one should look for constitutional or venereal diseases like tuberculosis, syphilis or chancroid. The cracks may be laterally placed if any of these are present.

Examination and Treatment

Injection treatment was attempted without much success in 1926 by Graham (87) and in 1929 by Gabriel (88). They used older, unsafe sclerosing solutions which were not as effective as our modern preparations. Today this troublesome condition, which is so often treated surgically by a wide excision of the anal ulcer with the underlying tissue, is readily cured by a modern injection method. The technique is easily learned and is performed in two separate stages.

The examination for the diagnosis of fissure in ano can be exactly the same as the first step in its actual treatment, therefore, it will be described here.

For diagnostic purposes I usually attempt the rectal examination without injection at first. For this a confident manner, continual reassurance and very gentle handling are necessary. Little strategems like asking the patient to relax, instructions to breathe deeply and relaxing verbal communication may suffice to control the patient's apprehension.

Wearing a finger cut or glove, the examining physician should attempt, in easy stages, to insert a finger into the anus using a mixture of two lubricating agents; 2% Nupercaine or Xylocaine ointment mixed with K-Y jelly. Once the finger succeeds in entering the anal canal, it is a simple matter to very gently dilate it and insert a lubricated anoscope (Brinkerhoff). The diagnosis becomes apparent during the dilation, and the fissure can be clearly identified as to location, size and depth.

If the spasm of the sphincter cannot be overcome by these simple measures, it will be necessary to anesthetize the fissure area and occasionally, the sphincter muscles. The patient is advised that he may feel a tiny pin prick as the first step.

Using a 2 or 3 c.c. syringe with a 30 gauge needle, the operator, after swabbing the area of injection near the ulcer, deposits several minums of 2% Xylocaine solution subcutaneously. This should be practically painless. It is followed by injecting the same anesthetic with a 22 gauge, 1½ inch needle, that has a bead on it to insure recovery if it breaks off during injection. The solution is injected as the needle is advanced on both sides of the fissure and also underneath it.

It is a matter of judgment as to how far away from the fissure wall, and the bottom of the fissure, the injection is made. One must leave sufficient tissue so that the resulting reaction will not unduly irritate the anal tissue adjoining the ulcer.

The anesthesia described may be needed to permit dilatation of the anal canal but it may also be a preliminary to actual sclerosing treatment. It may not be possible to inject the entire ulcer area in one step. The operator must then anesthetize as much as he can reach and step by step advance the needle a little further each time so that gradually the entire lesion will be treated. Usually the initial Xylocaine injection will produce enough anesthesia to permit at least partial insertion of the finger.

I have found that properly executed anesthetic injections are sufficient for a rapid cure in mild cases. For the more refractory conditions a long lasting anesthetic used to be available prior to FDA regulations in the United States. With the latter solution it was not necessary to use sclerotherapy for many cases of anal ulcer, as they would promptly close if kept relaxed for a week or more with long lasting anesthesia.

Refractory and advanced cases are now treated by sclerotherapy very successfully in the following manner. After the needle has been introduced to the proper length and depth of the fissure, and the Xylocaine has been properly distributed, it can be left in place for each injection. A syringe containing sodium morrhuate 2 to 5% is then substituted. If the needle has not been displaced by this manoeuver, it is a simple matter to deposit the sclerosing solution along the needle track as the syringe is withdrawn.

By repeating this procedure, the three areas mentioned above are safely bathed with the sclerosing agent during the withdrawal process.

It is important to distribute the chemical agent as evenly as possible so as to avoid pooling which might cause too much local irritation and possible necrosis of tissue. With practice an even flow of medication can be made.

The amount of solution and its type depends upon the size of the fissure and how advanced the pathology has become. In the average case, it is gratifying how .5 to 1 c.c. of 5% sodium morrhuate can cure a painful disabling fissure. It is only in the occasional advanced case that more treatments are necessary. These should be given at two week intervals. It is important to remember that we are dealing with infected delicate tissue that cannot tolerate too much chemical irritation. Indeed, it is rather remarkable that the above-mentioned dosage is so well tolerated and effective. Other solutions like Sotradecol and some of the older ones like Monolate can also be utilized.

In the occasional uncontrollably neurotic or hypersensitive patient, it may be necessary to inject most or all of the rectal sphincter for thorough relaxation prior to the sclerosing treatment. This also aids in the healing process because relaxation is one of the keys to a successful outcome.

It may not be necessary to inject the sidewalls in a small, early case. Merely placing .25 to .5 c.c. of 5% sodium morrhuate beneath the fissure may induce healing in many individuals.

The mechanism of the sclerosing action is unclear. The immediate aftereffect is induration and secondarily, fibrous tissue formation. This process may seal off the ulcerated skin from the underlying tissue thereby assisting the healing process. Also the edema following injection may close the ulcer opening by apposing its walls.

I have found this relatively simple technique to be uniformly successful and consider it the treatment of choice.

Chapter 18

■ PILONIDAL CYST

The treatment of pilonidal cyst, by the use of sclerosing solutions, was revived from an ancient technique described by Cutler and Zollinger in 1933 (89). I was prompted by their report to study this problem further, and this chapter is based on the successful new technique that was developed (Biegeleisen, H.) (90)

This disease was termed "pilonidal" by Hodges. The true meaning of the term is "nest of hair." These hairs may be found within the cystic dilatation which is present or may be seen protruding from the sinus openings. Those openings or depressions were considered a result of faulty fusion of the ectoderm in the sacrococcygeal region. Almost a third of newborn infants show a sinus in this area. While this often disappears with growth, about 4%, usually males, retain the defect.

In recent years, another viewpoint regarding the origin of this cyst has been proposed. It is considered by many that a pilonidal cyst simply develops from ingrowing hairs. To support this idea, it is pointed out that the lesion occurs at hairy points of repeated pressure, such as the coccygeal area.

A rather striking finding was reported in the literature when cases of pilondal cyst involving the back of the fingers in the interdigital webs were discovered in barbers. This supports the theory of constant pressure implanting hairs that continue to grow and form a cyst. Whether this is true or not, it is interesting to note that hairy cysts may form without congenital skin defects.

Whatever its origin, the pathology remains the same, and the typical cystic dilatation accompanied by sinuses forms.

The sinuses, single or multiple, vary in depth from a few millimeters to over an inch. The cystic dilatations may be present at any point of the sinus, but they usually occur at the end of the passage. In the frequent event of multiple sinuses, they may communicate with the same blind cystic pouch. Without infection, the only sign that might be noted would be one or more pinpoint openings in the skin from which long hairs protrude.

In the event of infection, the picture changes to that of a typical subcutaneous abscess with the difference that simple incision and drainage does not cure the condition. The basic hairy structure remains intact to resume its growth. The operator must not lose sight of this throughout the treatment.

It is interesting to note the ancient origin of sclerosing therapy and its recent revival. As early as 1829, Dzondi (91) treated fistulae of the neck by injection of Liquor Nitrici Hydrargyri. Since there is no evidence of its further use in the literature, this method for fistula must have proven discouraging.

The stimulus for the modern approach to this problem must be credited to the neurologic surgeons, Cutler and Zollinger. They noted that the linings of certain forms of gliomatous cysts could be hardened by the use of Carnoy's solution.

Modified Carnoy's Solution

Absolute Alcohol	– 6.
Chloroform	– 3.
Glacial Acetic Acid	– 1.
Ferric Chloride	–1.

The solution caused the cysts to become hardened and tougher, enabling the surgeon to remove them intact. In addition, hemostasis was obtained. Cutler and Zollinger seized upon these qualities in their treatment of cysts and fistulae.

I duplicated their method in pilonidal cyst with the thought that a simple sclerosing method might replace surgery. The procedure outlined by the above authors required incision and drainage of the abscess. Then Carnoy's solution was applied to the abscess cavity, and the cavity subsequently curetted. The cauterizing solution was also applied to the lining membrane of the sinus tracts. Cutler's method resulted in occasional cures. However, the solution advocated by him did not have sufficient sclerosing power to handle the majority of cases that came to my attention.

It was necessary to use a more potent sclerosing agent, and I found concentrated, fuming nitric acid to be an ideal solution for this technique. Despite its action as a powerful acid outside the body, it effectively destroyed the lining membrane painlessly and safely.

Often the first indication of a pilonidal cyst about the rectum, in the sacrococcygeal area, is a painful swelling which arises without any apparent cause. Patients are generally unaware of the existence of this cyst prior to inflammation or abscess formation. This brings them to the physician who makes the diagnosis which is based upon the discovery of the sinus openings. These abscesses must be treated by incision and drainage prior to any sclerosing treatment. All of the inflammation must subside completely before proceeding with the next step.

A problem may present itself after the patient gets complete relief by the incision and drainage. He will feel so well that it may be difficult to convince him that he still retains the cystic condition he had at the outset. In many cases, if further treatment is refused, another abscess will form within a matter of months or longer. It is important to make the patient realize that a permanent cure is impossible unless the pilonidal cyst is completely removed. Cases of healed abscesses and non-infected cases may be treated immediately by the technique that follows.

Technique

Special instruments are required in view of the fact that we are working in tiny areas. Some of these are so fine that it is necessary to use the same equipment that dentists use for root canal therapy and the technique is similar. The instruments include fine probes, curettes, and dental broaches. The latter is a tiny file which is mildly flexible so that it can be insinuated into a tortuous channel. The remainder of the equipment, which includes tiny curettes, malleable probes, and small applicators, is standard. Some of the instruments are also used in rhinology

In a simple case involving one sinus leading to a variable sized cyst, the operator will proceed as follows: Any protruding hairs are first extracted with forceps or small mosquito clamps. They come out readily because the roots of these hairs are not firmly attached as with normal hair. Then, a malleable probe is inserted through the skin opening and advanced until it finds the cystic sac. Often, the average probe will not enter the tiny skin opening, and finer equipment must be used. This consists of fine needles which have been deliberately dulled so that the points are ground away. Also, tiny dilators are inserted into the skin opening and, with pressure, the skin aperture is enlarged sufficiently to admit a probe. Probing is complete when the cystic enlargement of the sinus is revealed.

After the operator has outlined the location of the ducts and cystic sac, a modified Carnoy's solution is injected (92). This injection can also be done with a dull needle which is inserted into the sinus opening. The operator should inject enough solution to fill the sinus and sac. Curettage may be used immediately or on the next visit.

If the channel has been sufficiently dilated, it will now be possible to insert a tiny curette and scrape the lining of both sac and sinus. As this is done, hairs and lining membrane will both be pulled and scraped out of the duct openings. This manoeuver is continued until the operator is satisfied that the entire lining and its hairs have been removed. Sometimes the bolus or nest of hairs will come out in one mass. At other times it may be necessary to remove one or two hairs at a time. The operator must be satisfied that the condition has been completely curetted before proceeding further.

Preliminary skin anesthesia is advisable. Novocaine or Xylocaine solution, 2%, should be injected in the area or introduced through each sinus opening on a very fine cotton-tipped probe. The ducts and sac are now ready for the fuming nitric acid, which is the sclerosing agent. Again, a fine cotton-tipped probe is dipped into the acid, taking care that there are no excess drops, and the probe gently but firmly inserted through the sinus opening down to its complete length into the cyst cavity. As it traverses the sinus canal, it is rotated to bring the acid into contact with the entire circumference of the tract. It is very striking that the patient experiences no burning sensation with this apparently corrosive acid. Neither is there much residual after-pain. The patients are very comfortable with the nitric acid therapy.

Each case will present modifications of canals and central sacs which, together with the varying degrees of scar tissue found, will call for changes in the technique. Sometimes a channel may be curetted readily, and all the epithelial lining removed so the nitric acid will sclerose it successfully. In other cases, usually due to preceding infection, the lining membrane may be considerably thickened, so that when the epithelial layer is removed, layers of scar tissue will be found underneath it. This type of channel will not sclerose with the ordinary curettage-acid routine. It will be necessary to incise the channel and lay it open so effective curettage of the scar tissue may be done openly. This can now be followed by the application of the acid under direct observation with greater effectiveness.

Another obstacle to the usual blind probing and curettage will be found in extremely tortuous channels where even a flexible instrument cannot make the passage. Again, the operator must resort to a little additional minor skin surgery to lay the channel open in order to expose the end of the canal that cannot be reached by instrument. The acid treatment will follow under visual control.

Aside from the necessity for incising abscesses and difficult channels, the various kinds of cysts encountered will yield to the blind method outlined above. Treatments cannot be spaced too close to each other with this therapy, in order to allow time for healing to take place. The beneficial effects of the first treatment may be curetted and removed if another treatment follows too closely. Usually, one waits about a month before testing the effects of the treatment before repeating it. The author has found on occasion that when a channel is especially difficult to close, a longer waiting period of about three months may afford complete closure.

Testing should be performed in every case by gently attempting to insert a fine probe into the skin opening or openings, if they are multiple. This will determine whether the channels are closed. If the testing is done too soon, within one or two weeks, granulation tissue which may still be soft may be damaged or pierced by the examining probe. When the operator feels certain that mature healing has taken place, he will find that the probe cannot be pushed into the canals, and then the patient is considered cured.

It is important to exclude spina bifida before starting this treatment. In the latter condition, the spinal canal may be open, so that either infection or sclerosing solution can enter with varied results. In doubtful cases, x-ray visualization is warranted.

The results following sclerotherapy are often superior to surgery. Not only is the patient ambulatory throughout, but the results are less prone to failure. With the surgical approach, a large mass of tissue is excised "en-bloc" with the hope that all of the channels have been removed. Should any of them remain behind, it is possible for the entire cyst to reform. Some surgeons place the statistical recurrence rate at approximately 50%. The author has never had a failure in thirty-five years.

Case 1: Patient aged 16. Abscess in sacrococcygeal region for duration of one week. Under local anesthesia, the swelling was incised and the cavity packed with iodoform gauze. Three days later: abscessed cavity smaller, cleaned. Modified Carnoy's solution on a cotton-tipped applicator applied for 10 seconds. Two sinuses discovered leading into cavity. Two weeks later: cavity clean and almost closed. Three weeks later: three sinus openings located, curetted, treated with fuming nitric acid. Probe of the larger revealed it to be about two inches long. Long hairs removed upon curettage. Two weeks later: curettage and cauterization performed. One month later: one sinus closed, remaining two treated. One month later: largest sinus is still slightly open; curetted, and nitric acid applied. One month later: pilonidal cyst completely cured, sinus opening demonstrated firm scar tissue, probe cannot be inserted. One year later: no recurrence.

Case 2: Patient age 30, complaining of discharge on underwear, slight itching, discomfort in coccygeal region. Examination revealed pilonidal cyst, two sinuses, no infection. Sinuses were probed, sclerotic therapy instituted immediately. Preliminary probings were performed to determine length and direction of sinuses. First treatment instituted: modified Carnoy's solution injected through sinus opening using dull needle. Two weeks later: both sinuses curetted under Novocaine anesthesia with removal of numerous hairs and lining membrane. Fuming nitric acid applied on ordinary metal applicator tip, deeply into both sinuses. Sinus openings dressed, using small gauze pad containing boric acid ointment. Two weeks later: procedure repeated. One month later: attempted curettage, difficult to enter sinus tracts due to beginning obliteration. Probe with nitric acid admitted partly into each tract. Dry dressing applied. One month later: both sinuses completely closed. One year later: no recurrence.

Case 3: Patient, aged 33. Complained of itching, discharge in the sacrococcygeal region for several years. On examination pilonidal cyst with two sinus tracts was found. Probed to point of common intersection several times, modified Carnoy's solution injected. One week later: sinus tracts curetted using bent needle curette. Fuming nitric acid applied on probe into each. Two weeks later: another treatment administered. One month later: third treatment. Sinus openings smaller and gave difficulty in probing. One month later: both sinus openings firmly closed, patient discharged. Six months later: identical findings.

Chapter 19

■ HYDROCELE

A hydrocele is a circumscribed collection of fluid in a sac, usually within the scrotum. It may arise in various ways and be found in different locations in the scrotum. Most commonly it forms in the tunica vaginalis of the testicle or along the spermatic cord. In the congenital type it forms in the unobliterated canal between the peritoneal cavity and the tunica vaginalis. It may be present in hernial sacs or even in connection with the round ligament of the female. Very seldom are two hydroceles found at the same time.

It is easily recognized by palpation and, if necessary, by transillumination. They are usually amenable to injection treatment with the exceptions noted below.

Technique

The first step is to tap the sac using a 19-20 gauge needle, 1½ to 2 inches long. It is not always necessary to anesthetize the skin as the insertion of the tapping needle may be made rather painlessly by a quick thrust through the skin and tunica vaginalis. The operator may, however, prefer to treat the skin first by raising an intradermal wheal with a 27 guage needle, using 1% Xylocaine. Care must be taken on entering the sac not to injure the testicle, but this is easily avoided especially in large effusions. It may be helpful to transilluminate again during this procedure it there is any doubt at all, but experienced operators don't find this necessary.

Caution must be observed not to displace the needle tip while draining the hydrocele. As the sac shrinks in size during the emptying process, the needle has a tendency to be pulled in by the contracting sac. Therefore, while the hand holding the syringe is extracting the fluid, the other hand must manually keep the needle in place within the shrinking sac. This manoeuver must be performed while guarding the testicle. Once learned, it can readily be duplicated.

The fluid is withdrawn by the syringe and emptied into an emesis basin or glass graduate to be measured and studied. It may be analyzed for cells or bacteria if cloudy. The rather rare instances of malignancy, tuberculosis, or infection may thus be ruled out. The amount of sclerosing solution used will depend upon the quantity of fluid withdrawn. Occasionally it may be blood tinged if there has been some trauma to the tissues. This need cause no alarm as any slight hemorrhage is self-limited. It is usually controlled by the contraction of the sac and the coagulating action of the sclerosing solution.

The next step is the injection of the sclerosing solution. However, I have found it advisable, especially in sensitive individuals, to make a preliminary injection of 1 or 2 c.c. of 2% Procaine or Xylocaine solution into the sac. This will eliminate the occasional mild shock reaction due to the initial irritation of the sclerosing fluid acting on the testicular membranes.

There is a choice of sclerosing solution depending upon the age of the patient, the size of the hydrocele, the thickness of its wall and the sensitivity of the patient. For example, I would treat an infant or child up to puberty with a very mild solution like sodium morrhuate, using anywhere from 2 minims to 2 c.c. At the age of 2 years, I would start with .5 c.c. in an average case.

With adults, where the tissues are less delicate and more mature, or even thickened, I use 1 to 2 c.c. of quinine and urethane solution. It is also possible to use sodium morrhuate and Sotradecol 3% in quantities from 1 to 5 c.c. depending upon the size of the sac and the fluid within. It is better to aim at mild reactions. To ensure such a reaction in early hydroceles it may be wise to employ 1 to 2 c.c. of a 1% Sotradecol solution.

The reaction following injection must be clearly understood not only by the doctor but by the patient, as well. Following the treatment, the hydrocele sac will swell up again within a few days to its original size or even larger. The patient may express disappointment and apprehension, as the hydrocele now seems not only to have returned but is tender, warm and quite hard. The patient must be reassured that it will gradually subside until there is no trace of the hydrocele left.

It is advisable that the patient wears either a suspensory or jock strap to support the hardened, tender sac until the reaction subsides. The tenderness may be relieved by using ice bags or cold compresses for the first few days. The patient may also take ordinary analgesics like aspirin or more effective preparations.

The average case of adult hydrocele will be moderately sensitive for perhaps five days and will usually subside within four weeks. Smaller cases and younger individuals will heal in a few weeks. However, I have had neglected cases in older men with large sacs who have taken as much as three months for complete subsidence. In all cases, if the patient will follow the doctor's counsel and not be unduly alarmed by the initial swelling, there will be a most gratifying and almost magical disappearance of the hydrocele sac to everyone's satisfaction.

Sometimes the operator will need great power of persuasion to convince the patient that the treatment has not made him worse because the painless enlargement of his hydrocele has become converted into a hot, tender, hard mass. It must be explained that this is merely the normal reaction of tissue induration and that it will gradually be absorbed day by day until it is completely gone. It is entirely possible for an apprehensive individual at this juncture to consult another practitioner who may not be aware of the mode of action with this therapy. Interference at this point by further injection or surgery may have serious consequences and should be strictly forbidden. After a few days of patience the picture will dramatically improve and healing from then on will be smooth.

I prefer the quinine solution if there is no history of cinchonism because it produces less initial inflammation with less swelling and more rapid healing than do fatty acid preparations like sodium morrhuate. However, each operator may have his own preferences depending upon his experience and skill.

When contrasted with the radical *bottle operation* in which the scrotum is opened, the tunica vaginalis inverted and sutured into place with the attendant morbidity and possible complications, the injection procedure becomes a preferable alternative.

When properly executed, after healing has taken place, there is usually no trace left of the original hydrocele sac or mass. There are no skin scars. This technique, with its often perfect results, is an outstanding example of the value of sclerotherapy.

Chapter 20

▪ VARICOCELE

Varicocele is a varicose condition of the veins along the spermatic cord in the scrotum. It has been compared to a "bag of worms" when felt by the examiner's hand. It is treated like varicose veins on the lower extremity with one important difference. That is the special technique described below, which requires considerable manual dexterity because these blood vessels are not fixed, but float rather freely within the scrotum.

The varicocele may be unilateral or bilateral. The former is much more frequent. There can be an amazing variation in size depending upon the number of veins involved. In a minor case there may be only a few varicosities that have enlarged while major cases can form masses of remarkable size. The gross appearance of these advanced cases may resemble a scrotal hernia.

To differentiate between a varicocele, hydrocele, or hernia, it may be helpful at times to transilluminate the enlargement. Thus, light coming through the liquid contents of a sac will indicate the presence of a hydrocele. A hernia will not transmit the examining light at all while in a varicocele the opacity of the mass is not as pronounced as in hernia.

Palpation of the scrotum will often suffice to make the diagnosis without an examining light. Hydrocele will be felt as a fluctuating liquid cyst of fixed size. A hernia on coughing will transmit the characteristic expansile intestinal impulse. In varicocele there is no better description than the resemblance to the bag of worms mentioned previously. Once this is felt by the operator in a typical case, it will never be forgotten.

The solutions used are the same as those in ordinary varicose veins. Here, too, the physician should aim for reactions on the milder side. Fortunately it is not necessary to inject each vein separately. There is frequent communication between them and injecting any of the larger ones may suffice to obliterate a large part, or indeed, all of the clustered blood vessels.

In this technique the patient stands on the floor while the operator is seated on a stool in front of him. The object is to try transfixing one of the more prominent veins by holding the varicose mass with one hand while injecting with the other. With some practice the operator will learn to hold the slippery group of veins with one hand in such a manner as to keep them contained, while at the same time tightening the skin around them. He should pick a prominent vein in the varicocele cluster when attempting the injection.

Having thus immobilized the veins, the operator, using a 2 to 5 c.c. glass syringe with a 23 or 21 gauge 1½ inch needle, should attempt to enter the vein lumen by a sharp thrust. Sometimes with a nervous patient it may be necessary to precede this injection by raising a skin wheal with 1% Xylocaine at the site of entry. More often the skin and vein can both be penetrated simultaneously without the anesthetic if the needle point is sharp and its thrust is quickly performed as mentioned above.

This technique requires special handling for the timorous patient. The physician must calmly reassure any patient who may be apprehensive regarding a genital injection that there is little, if any, pain involved. It does not matter which vein is entered, as stated above, because they often communicate. Sometimes the operator aims for one blood vessel and accidentally finds another, which usually serves the same purpose. Proof of entry is the appearance of blood on aspiration. One must never inject a varicocele perivascularly.

From 1 to 5 c.c. of the following solutions may be used depending upon the size of the mass and the number of veins. In order of increasing effectiveness they are: sodium morrhuate, Sotradecol, quinine, and urethane. One should not exceed 2 c.c. of quinine because of the side effects of cinchonism. It may require several injections the same day or perhaps several visits to completely sclerose the entire varicocele.

Following the treatment the varicocele may swell to present an even greater mass than the original one. If the operator is extremely dextrous or fortunate enough to find a vein with the patient lying down to perform an empty vein injection (see Chapter V for technique), he may avoid the post-injection swelling to a considerable degree but it is often impractical to achieve this.

The patient is instructed to wear a firm suspensory or jock-strap until the sclerosed veins, which now form a definite lump within the scrotum, subside to normalcy. He must be strongly cautioned not to be alarmed at the swelling or pain that follows the treatment as this is a perfectly normal response that will always subside.

For immediate pain or swelling, cold compresses, two or three times a day, are effective. An ice bag may be applied directly on the suspensory. Sometimes anti-inflammatory drugs like Butazolidin or others may be useful in ameliorating the reaction. Healing may take anywhere from one to several weeks but subsidence is the rule.

When concluded the result is remarkable as there will be no trace of the pre-existing condition and no visible evidence of any treatment. Sclerotherapy in this condition has proven superior to surgery with its risk of complications. In trained hands, this is the treatment of choice.

Chapter 21

▪ BURSITIS

Bursae are little cushions in the musculoskeletal system which contain a secretion of synovial fluid. This is physically and chemically the same as joint fluid because the bursa is lined with a membrane similar to synovial membrane. The sac is covered outwardly by fibrous tissue.

Bursal sacs are usually monolocular containing only a single cavity but occasionally may develop membranes dividing them into two or more little chambers. There are dozens of scattered bussae which are not important enough to be named. Only a few of practical importance like the prepatellar, acromial and olecranon have received specific names.

Adventitious bursae may develop at any time in response to the need for lubrication at all points where sufficient friction or motion exists. They usually are found where tendons and muscles work around corners and at points where muscles cross in opposite directions. Also they are seen between areas where skin over bone requires lubrication. Bursae operate as would any fluid sac placed between two opposing pressures so that, with a certain amount of play, there will be a gliding, lubricated motion which is made possible by a limited wrinkling and tightening of one or both walls.

Once formed, bursae can be the site of local inflammation due to injury with resulting infection. They can also be affected by systemic disorders. Sometimes a large pus sac may form as in infected "house-maid's knee."

Deeply placed bursae may also become inflamed as the result of chronic strain or, perhaps, an inflammatory condition in the surrounding tissues. Here, with the hyperemia produced, an effusion may distend the closed sac that can be agonizingly painful.

The synovial sacs and the fibrous outer walls are subject to all the ills that afflict the rest of the body. Thus specific diseases and tumor formation are possibilities to be borne in mind for differential diagnosis. Gout is an outstanding example of a metabolic disease with a predilection for bursal involvement. Here crystals of sodium urate may be found within the bursae, sometimes in great quantities. Occasionally, these gouty accumulations will rupture into the tissues or become infected.

Calcific deposits are different and are the bane of chronic or advanced bursitis. They are most common in the shoulder in association with subdeltoid or subacromial bursitis. Here there is a tendon cuff or sheath which is the seat of deposits of calcium salts that are not always within the sac, as commonly supposed. Sometimes, the mass of calcium may rupture out of the tendon sheath into the bursa. In grossly advanced cases, a binding process results gluing the bursa, cuff tendon and muscle together to cause restriction of motion and a "frozen shoulder." Calcific deposits of the rotator tendons may occur which, even here, may not cause involvement within the sac. This kind of calcification does not necessarily produce any pain, but more often, the converse is true and chronic pain results.

In the chronic stage, the lining is subject to the pathologic condition of hypertrophic villus formation causing not only pain on pressure but a crackling sensation on manual manipulation of the sac. These conditions may arise in anatomical as well as adventitious locations and the treatment described is the same for both. It is vital to decide whether or not the bursa is infected prior to sclerotherapy. In the event that infection has taken place, one must not inject. The infection or suppuration, if it is that far advanced, must be first drained and eliminated before injection treatment can be considered. Usually the bursae will reform after drainage and if the fluid is clear the injection treatment which has been postponed may now be started. This rule applies to all cases of bursitis.

Pre-Patellar Bursitis (Housemaid's Knee)

As an example of injection treatment for bursitis the procedure for housemaid's knee will be described.

This condition, a pre-patellar bursitis, was the first type I dealt with in the early days of sclerosing therapy and its technique, which follows, has not changed.

To confirm the diagnosis one can show the transparency of the contained fluid by transillumination. Transmission of the light will indicate a fluid sac which is ready for treatment.

Technique

After preliminary skin anesthesia by raising a wheal of Procaine 1%, tapping is first performed using a 17 to 19 gauge, 2- or 3-inch needle. This is inserted below or to the side of the patella, entering the large distended bursa underneath the kneecap. If the accumulation of fluid is extensive enough, boundaries will be lost and the most dependent bulge can be the site of tapping and subsequent injection.

The bursal swelling is emptied of clear fluid and the amount removed is measured. Some minor bleeding from small blood vessels in the cyst walls may be disregarded.

Depending upon the sensitivity of the patient and the amount of fluid involved, the sac is either injected directly with the sclerosing fluid, or a few c.c. of Procaine or Xylocaine is first introduced prior to the actual irritating solution. I cannot prescribe any rule for this determination as it is a matter of judgment for the individual operator.

With the average pre-patellar bursitis 1 to 5 c.c. of 5% sodium morrhuate will suffice to sclerose this kind of a case. I have extracted anywhere from 5 to 20 c.c. or more, of synovial fluid from cases of this type. The size of the injection, therefore, would roughly be 1 c.c. of sclerosing agent for every 4 to 5 c.c. of withdrawn fluid. The injection is covered by a gauze dressing over which the operator wraps a three inch elastic bandage. This may be of easily removable type or one made of elastic adhesive (Elastoplast).*

Following this injection, the reaction that is anticipated must be carefully explained to the patient. After several hours, or by the end of the day, the bursa and the area surrounding it, due to the chemical irritation, will swell perhaps to its former size or sometimes even larger. This will be accompanied by some warmth, considerable tenderness and a hardening of the tissues. The mass thus formed will certainly frighten the uninformed patient leading him to think that he is getting worse. There have been instances where, at this point, a frightened patient will go to another physician and here is where serious trouble may occur.

Confronted with such a tumor mass, the second doctor consulted, may assume that an infection has taken place. He may even incise the mass and really start an infection that would normally never take place.

The reaction following treatment, if left to heal according to the operator's instructions, will not present any difficulty. These orders are to keep an elastic bandage 3 to 4 inches in width wrapped around the knee joint comfortably but firmly so that some flexion of the knee is possible without much pain. If needed an ice bag or cold pack may be placed over the injected bursa or right on top of the elastic bandage. This cooling action can be maintained

---

* BDF Beiersdorf Inc. So. Norwalk, Conn. 06854

for 15 minutes several times during the first day. The usual simple analgesic tablets may also be taken by the patient if so disposed.

The inflamed mass will always subside day by day until complete subsidence takes place. This means that the walls of the sac have adhered, fibrosed and for all practical purposes, disappeared. There should be no sign of a bursa afterwards. In properly treated cases, this is far superior to the alternative method of surgical removal with its attendant external scarring and possible injury to the adjoining knee joint tissues.

This picture of a treatment for a classical case of pre-patella bursitis is similar to that which follows the other types of sclerotherapy for bursal sacs. In other locations conditions are met with that require altered techniques and often other solutions. These include Sotradecol 3% and Sylnasol. The Sotradecol solution, which is the more potent sclerosing agent, can be used in smaller quantities.

Generallly speaking, any bursa that has an effusion and is not infected is suitable for sclerosing therapy. The operator must have a knowledge of the anatomy in the area he is treating. The bursa must show definite fluctuation and has to be within reach of the needle for this technique.

When these conditions are fulfilled, the effusion is tapped and the amount of fluid withdrawn is measured. For small bursae, where only a few minims are extracted, a correspondingly small dosage of sclerosing agent is injected. The effectiveness of sclerotherapy under these conditions is consistently good. Unfortunately, most cases of bursitis do not present themselves with such a ripe and easily located sac. The usual type of bursitis that comes to the doctor's attention is the chronic, dry type sometimes containing calcium or other deposits.

The dry types of inflamed bursae, either in the early chronic or later intractible stages, are often one of the most refractory conditions to treat by any method. They form a group of painful afflictions which sometimes exhibit exquisite tenderness and often defy conventional treatments. These include x-ray therapy, spraying with ethyl chloride, and injections, into the area, of Xylocaine with or without steroids.

Several techniques are employed to handle calcium deposits. Needling with anesthetic solutions mentioned above sometimes breaks up the calcium accumulations which are aspirated with large bore needles or subsequently absorbed by the tissues. Still another method, if the operator can find his way into the bursal sac, is to wash it out using normal saline solution. Occasionally this, too, may break up the deposits which are then aspirated or allowed to remain for natural absorption.

None of these methods can be relied upon to handle all the dry cases. They properly do not fall within the scope of this book on sclerotherapy. However, it is possible to use sclerosing methods in a special way which I developed in 1957 and which I termed "provocative" sclerotherapy.

Provocative Sclerotherapy

Ordinary sclerosing procedures cannot be employed where there is no discernable sac that can be identified. To overcome this handicap, I employ a mild sclerosing agent like .25 or .5 strength, sodium morrhuate solution to irritate but not sclerose the elusive bursal sac. The response to a provocative injection, if successful, is an effusion into the bursa. This identifies and outlines the sac.

Chronic cases of dry bursitis which do not respond to conventional treatment and may be causing severe pain can thus be converted into acute flare-ups of bursitis with effusion. If this occurs, the next step is to tap the sac and inject directly into the now easily outlined bursa with 5% sodium morrhuate or other sclerosing agents. Any dry bursa that responds to provocative injection can therefore be satisfactorily treated by sclerotherapy.

This technique is eminently suitable for olecranon bursitis where the bursa and its calcific deposits, if present, is easily palpable under the skin, and the provocative injection can then be accurately placed into the bursal sac or area. Sometimes even injecting the area provocatively will cause a new bursal effusion that thereby becomes amenable to injection treatment.

Superficial bursae in the region of the Achilles tendon, bunion area and other accessible points on the foot are also susceptible to this type of provocative treatment. Where the shoulder bursae are more deeply placed, as in the sub-acromial or sub-deltoid groups, this technique is more difficult to apply.

Sclerotherapy, by irritating and injuring the sac lining, stimulates the growth of fibrous tissue to cause adhesions between opposing layers of the sac. This fibrotic process removes the sac effectively with no visible scarring. Any crystalline deposits around the sac will no longer press on a sensitive area. This eliminates the painful syndrome of bursitis.

More studies in the area of chronic bursitis are needed to further refine the technique. In my experience, it has been the answer to some very troublesome cases without resorting to surgery. For ordinary bursitis with effusion, there is no question in my mind that simple aspiration followed by sclerotherapy is the preferred treatment.

Chapter 22

■ GANGLION

The common ganglion on the dorsum of the wrist is easily recognizable by most practitioners. This cystic tumor is part of a group of growths derived from cells destined to form the membranes, capsules and ligaments of joints. They are, in fact, tumors of synovial cell origin and might be called synoviomas.

Ganglia are frequent tumors of the human body. Their origin has been disputed, but most believe that it is due to trauma because it recurs so frequently in people who subject their limbs to repeated motion. Thus pianists, violinists, typists or others who use the hands for long periods of detailed coordinated work are subject to this disorder.

However, there are many individuals who develop ganglia who do not have this kind of repetitive occupation. This led, years ago, to another theory of its origin. Many surgeons considered the condition a herniation of the synovial sheath through a tiny opening in the capsule of a joint. Actual communication has never been demonstrated but the theory is still held.

As a result of my work with injection treatment in other fascial tissues, I feel that the ganglia I have treated were often due to tissue degeneration. This view is supported by the theory of inherited fascial weakness (93). It seems plausible for the fascial structures, in this case the synovial sheaths and capsules, to become weakened or relaxed making them prone to degeneration. A similar pathology occurs in the ligaments of the spine where they are also subject to demonstrable degenerative changes (Chapter 23).

Ganglia are most frequently found in association with the wrist and finger joints. They are also seen around the ankle joint. However, they may occur in connection with any joint capsule where weakening of the capsular contents can cause the formation of a cyst containing the characteristic gelatinous fluid within it.

In the region of the hand, ganglia may be dorsal, carpal, or volarcarpal. They may also be seen over the flexor tendons of the fingers, usually the proximal phalanges of the index, middle, and ring fingers. In these last locations, the little cysts feel so hard as to be confused with sesamoid bones.

Attempts at treatment for ganglia have a long history in medicine. The time honored method of hitting the tumor with a book in order to smash it, usually the Bible, have rarely been successful. The procedure is quite painful and is usually followed by recurrence. Aspiration of the contents of the sac is also not curative despite the many attempts that have been made with this method.

Surgery is the most commonly used method for ganglia but it is not a simple procedure. The areas involved are difficult to operate in without complications. In operating on a ganglion, it is important not only to remove the intact cyst, but also all of the basal tissue from which it springs. Recurrences follow if any basal tissue is left behind, and it is often difficult to distinguish ganglionic tissue from the normal joint capsule. As the difficulty of a cure increases with surgery, so does the potential for joint damage if a second operation is necessary. Also, the hazard of keloid formation must be considered. This is especially troublesome and unsightly on the volar aspect of the fingers. None of these problems exist with the injection method.

Before starting the injection method it is useful to make the ganglion more distinct by flexing the joint that it is connected with. Thus, in the case of a dorsocarpal ganglion, flexing the hand will outline the enlargement more distinctly. One should not attempt to treat a ganglion that is not large enough to receive at least 3 minims of solution because it will leak out immediately after the injection, and there will be no sclerosing action possible. The smaller cysts must be left alone until they enlarge. Sometimes a provocative injection of a relatively weak sclerosing agent like 5% sodium morrhuate may be injected to enlarge cyst by chemical irritation. Usually time will cause enlargement. Having decided that the cyst is large enough for treatment, the technique is as follows.

Technique

After preliminary local anesthesia, the sac must first be emptied with a large bore needle (17 to 19 gauge) to remove the gelatinous contents. Keeping the needle in place, the sclerosing solution is now injected so as to distend the sac. Only in large ganglia is this method altered. Here enough solution to irritate the walls is injected and the sac is outlined but distention is not attempted.

A mild sclerosing solution like 5% sodium morrhuate can be attempted for smaller ganglia because occasionally this will be sufficient to effect a cure. The determining factor in selecting the proper sclerosing agent, however,

Table 2
ZINC AND PHENOL STOCK SOLUTIONS

*1. Cloudy Stock Solution

Zinc Sulphate	4 gm
Phenol	24 gm
Glycerine	16 gm
Aqua q.s. ad	100 gm

2. 2-Ply Solution

Zinc Sulphate	8 gm
Phenol	12 gm
Glycerine	20 gm
Aqua a.s. ad	100 gm

3. 3-Ply Solution

Zinc Sulphate	12 gm
Phenol	12 gm
Glycerine	22 gm
Aqua a.s. ad	100 gm

4. 4-Ply Solution

Zinc Sulphate	16 gm
Phenol	12 gm
Glycerine	24 gm
Aqua a.s. ad	100 gm

* Note: Do not inject more than 1 c.c. of any of these stock mixtures at a time to avoid Phenol toxicity.

is not only the size of the tumor but also the thickness and degree of fibrosis of the wall itself. In a newly formed ganglion, if the patient is seen early enough, the walls of the sac will be thinner and more tender so that milder irritation may destroy the lining effectually and the walls will coalesce to form a flattened scar.

I have found it necessary, in most ganglion cases, to inject the same kind of fascial obliterants required for the treatment of inguinal hernia. This is not surprising because the type of tissue involved in both these instances is of the same tough, sinewy type.

I have found it useful to prepare stock mixtures containing phenol, glycerine, and zinc sulphate, in four strengths, for hernial obliteration, which are also suitable for ganglia (see Table 2). It will be noted that the first one is a cloudy, shake mixture, and is the usual formula for most cases. Increasing the glycerine component up to 24 gm converts the formula to a clear solution. The sclerosing power depends largely upon the proportion of zinc sulphate in the mixture. The cloudy solutions have delayed action, while the clear ones act more immediately and are more potent sclerosing agents for fascia. Thus, the operator can modify the potency of the stock solutions by altering the zinc concentration, or by adding glycerine to make the mixture clear. However, phenol, in the clear mixtures remains at 12 gm, to avoid toxicity.

In using the above solution, the operator must be certain that he has preceded the injection by employing a few c.c. of 2% Xylocaine or more as needed to flush out the sac. This anesthetic solution should be aspirated before injecting the zinc mixture. Normally, the sclerosing mixture will not irritate too much and will be well borne by the patient's tissues. Whatever is injected must be localized in the sac by placing an appropriate gauze sponge over it to retain the solution while it is absorbed.

The average ganglion of the wrist will be found to contain 1 to 3 c.c. of the gelatinous component which is aspirated by a syringe assisted by manual pressure and wrist flexion to empty it as completely as possible. In such an average case, the operator will inject approximately .5 to 1 c.c. of appropriately diluted sclerosing mixture (Table 2) and seal the opening with a gauze ball sponge. It may be useful to apply a cold compress containing ice cubes to reduce the immediate inflammatory response if needed.

With sensitive individuals, I leave some of the Xylocaine solution in the sac which has been previously injected and then introduce the sclerosing mixture to join it. This will considerably reduce the impact of the zinc sulfate action. For larger ganglia containing more than 3 c.c. of tumor jelly, some experience is needed to judge the potency of the injection.

I would suggest that before attempting to use large doses of a powerful sclerosing agent, one should make a preliminary test with perhaps 1 to 2 c.c. of a milder agent. If insufficient to sclerose the sac, the operator can then continue up the scale of increasing potency by injecting the shake mixture of zinc-phenol solution. From this he can use 1- or 2-ply clear zinc-phenol solution. It will be noted that the mixtures containing 2- and 3-ply zinc sulfate do not run the phenol concentration up, which remains at 12 gm per 100 c.c. The sclerosing action depends largely on the concentration of zinc sulphate in the stock mixtures. It is very important to note that one cannot use more than 1 c.c. of any stock solution at a time for any patient because of the phenol content.

If a larger amount of sclerosing fluid is needed for large ganglia, it may be made by adding sufficient anesthetic solution to build up the total volume. This is no problem because one can add 5 to 10 c.c. of 1 or 2% Xylocaine to the proper basic stock zinc phenol mixture so as to get a total volume of 5 to 10 c.c. The operator will be able to augment the sclerosing power and volume of the solutions required in each case. For instance, one can add 5 to 10 c.c. of 1 or 2% Procaine or Xylocaine to 1 c.c. of a 3-ply mixture to render a maximum sclerosing impact safely to a large, thick walled cyst. There is sufficient elasticity within these limits to make a mixture that will sclerose any ganglion. Sometimes a treatment may have to be repeated one or two times to completely efface a stubborn case.

When compared to surgical incision of ganglia connected with important joints like the wrist or ankle joint, sclerotherapy is much less traumatic to the joint tissues. A firm fibrosis obtained by the injection of the zinc phenol mixture produces an ideal result without hospitalization. Furthermore, there is no scar remaining, and in my experience, the results have been permanent. Patients who have had previous unsuccessful surgery are quick to appreciate the advantages of the injection method. It should be considered as a useful substitute for surgery.

Chapter 23

▪ LOW BACK SYNDROME

The subject of low back disorders has been the most maligned, confused and controversial chapter in the whole area of modern medicine. As a result, a maze of contradictions developed which has given rise to cults outside of medicine and splinter groups within its ranks. Each group claims it has the answer for this ancient disorder of mankind.

Organized medicine is not without blame for this confusion. It has revered with unwarranted veneration the hoary concept that the sacroiliac joint is the strongest in the body and is almost indestructible under ordinary conditions. This belief has been handed down without question from book to book.

Most physicians believe that injury to this joint and its large ligaments can occur only as the result of unusual crushing trauma. This erroneous concept has caused more suffering and disability, produced more wrong diagnosis, and created more hostility than any other in medicine. For, as shall be seen, the sacrum and its attached ligaments is the seat of a whole series of ligamentous disorders which have been relatively neglected for centuries on account of this belief.

When Mixter and Barr (94) in 1934 recognized that intervertebral disc injury or disease caused herniation of the nucleus pulposus, it was the first forward step in the treatment of low back disorders in modern times. This is an unquestionable clinical syndrome but is responsible for only a minor proportion of back conditions. Unfortunately, the exaggeration of the incidence and importance of herniated discs in low back disorders has resulted in overzealous and unwarranted surgery. Barr himself wrote that too many operations were being performed for back conditions and that these caused permanent damage. It is only fairly recently that orthopedists have become aware of the fact that back surgery destroys important ligaments and bony attachments that are needed for support. Due to the many failures, a changed viewpoint has resulted.

Later, Ghormley (95), Gardner (96), and Scuderi (97) brought attention to the strained sacroiliac joint as a source of symptoms and warned against undue reliance on disc surgery and spinal fusion. Early workers in sclerotherapy for ligament disability have long pointed out that only a small percentage of low back cases have ruptured discs that require surgery. Over 90% have ligament disability that can be corrected, and not just relieved, by injection treatment. Even true disc cases with definite lasting neurologic symptoms, in addition, usually have associated ligament relaxation, which may require post-operative strengthening by injections.

The literature does not disclose the etiology of ligamentous breakdown. That this is still a mystery is not surprising when simple degenerations like cloudy swelling are still not completely understood by pathologists. The supposedly impregnable sacroiliac ligament may often become the seat of softening or degeneration unexpectedly. Since the human skeleton depends upon the integrity of this structure for its upright posture, weakening and softening of it, with concommitant relaxation, is a serious disease. I have pointed out in Chapter 15 that fascial weakness can affect this as well as other ligaments. There is no doubt that frequent associations between the various kinds of ligament disorders is commonplace. I have found in my experience that it is rather rare for patients to exhibit only one fascial weakness. The genetic influences are apparent to the experienced operators in the field.

It is a moot question as to which comes first, the inherited weakness causing degeneration of the tissue or, conversely, tissue degeneration ending in ligament relaxation. There has been hardly any work on this important question. More investigation is urgently needed.

History

Writing in *Clinical Medicine and Surgery* in April, 1940 (98), I drew attention to the value of injecting sclerosing solutions in the treatment of hypermobile joints. I suggested then that Sylnasol be injected to promote adhesions in the area of capsular and articular ligaments to produce joint fixation.

At this time, I was also contemplating the use of sclerosing solutions for low back conditions including herniated disc. After considerable cadaver dissections, I worked out a series of injection angles using a 4 inch, 20 guage needle or a 3½ inch, 19 gauge needle, aimed at injections into the disc itself for the purpose of solidifying and sclerosing the disc material. This was not pursued because Gedney (99) and Hackett (100) were beginning to extend the scope of sclerotherapy in low back disorders by injecting the supporting ligaments instead. To digress for a moment, it is interesting to note that one of the more modern techniques for treating herniated discs is a return to the actual intra-disc injection using Chymopapain, which is a tissue digestant. This achieves digestion and absorption of the entire nucleus pulposis. Favorable results have been reported by a series of workers (101).

The three pioneer workers mentioned above were soon able to demonstrate the effectiveness of sclerotherapy for ligament relaxation. The fibrosis that developed was similar to the familiar responses obtained in other parts of the body. This work launched a whole new clinical extension of the art of sclerotherapy as applied to the back.

Hackett, a student of Head, the British neurologist, brought to America the first clear concept of referred pain arising from irritation along the spinal nerves of the spinal cord. This newer knowledge helped to form the basis of modern sclerotherapy for low back disorders.

It was now possible to explain and treat the varied syndromes of pain in the lower extremities, that were referred from the ligaments supporting the vertebral column and pelvis. It has also become possible to identify the ligaments causing the referred pain because the operator was now able to reproduce the pain by needling the suspected ligament. This made the technique a scientific process.

Early Technique and Solutions

As mentioned above, early workers like Gedney (102) in 1937 began the treatment of weakened sacroiliacs by the use of Sylnasol. His original technique involved injecting the lateral reflection of the anterior spinal ligament. He originally intended this to be helpful in cases of herniated disc. This was reported in "Disc Syndrome" in 1951.

Techniques were developed next for injecting the sacroiliac and lumbar ligaments. Sylnasol was used in this early phase. Unfortunately, it convulsed the patients with severe after-pain lasting up to 24 hours or more. Cold applications did not relieve this severe spasm. Neither did combining the Sylnasol solution with Pontocaine 0.15% or other local anesthetics. Following the treatment, each patient received tablets of Demerol, 50 mg, which did not subdue the painful reaction.

Progression of Solutions

There was obviously a need for improved solutions for this condition. The first step was to eliminate the disability and severe pain following the injection treatment with fatty-acid solutions like sodium morrhuate and Sylnasol. In order to achieve this quickly, and based upon my experience with fascial sclerosants in the treatment of ganglion and herniae, patients with low back conditions involving the sacroiliac and pelvic ligaments were treated with zinc phenol mixtures, as outlined elsewhere. This change stopped the agonizing after-pains which previously followed Sylnasol therapy.

Only local discomfort which lasted a few hours followed this new injection. It was easily controlled by either hot or cold applications, with a minimum of sedative therapy. Many patients required no other treatment while others were relieved easily by an aspirin tablet.

None of the patients receiving this solution had any remaining local discomfort on the following day and were able to resume their usual activities. This was in sharp contrast to the disabling reactions following Sylnasol therapy.

At this juncture leaders in sclerotherapy for back disorders turned to zinc phenol therapy as the next phase in solutions for its treatment. My interest in proposing these mixtures of zinc and phenol was to avoid primarily the after-pain. At the same time, the mixture was a more efficient fascial sclerosant and produced quick results in symptomatic improvement.

Referring to the formulae listed below, there are six mixtures of stock solutions in varying strengths. These are the same as recommended for ganglion and hernia treatment in Chapters 22 and 24. They are, however, used in a different fashion.

While the basic stock solution, which is a cloudy, shake mixture (Formula 1), can be used in its concentrated form without dilution for hernial sclerosis, it is usually diluted 1 to 10 with 1% Xylocaine for sacroiliac ligament therapy. If the operator desires to work with this type of mixture, he may decide to use the stronger formulae for resistant cases. For this reason the four different formulae mentioned in Chapter 22 are repeated here for quick reference, with two additions.

In general, the cloudy, shake mixtures are more slowly absorbed and have less immediate sclerosing power, while the clear solutions will have greater and more immediate impact because of their quicker absorption. In no instance can more than 1 c.c. of stock solution be used prior to dilution for injection treatment because of the phenol content of these formulae. However, up to 10 c.c. of total mixture can be injected to cover several areas of ligament treatment.

It will be noticed that the various formulae differ chiefly by virtue of the zinc sulphate concentration which is the agent chiefly responsible for its sclerosing action. Thus, zinc sulphate is present in the following concentrations: 4, 8, 12, and 16%. The clarity of the mixture depends upon the amount

Table 3
STOCK SOLUTIONS (BIEGELEISEN)

Cloudy, shake		Clear	
Basic			
1. $ZnSO_4$	4	3. $ZnSO_4$	4
Phenol	24	Phenol	24
Glycerine	16	Glycerine	24
Aq. q.s.	100	Aq. q.s.	100
2-ply			
2. $ZnSO_4$	8	4. $ZnSO_4$	8
Phenol	12	Phenol	12
Glycerine	8	Glycerine	24
Aq. q.s.	100	Aq. q.s.	100
3-ply			
		5. $ZnSO_4$	12
		Phenol	12
		Glycerine	24
		Aq. q.s.	100
4-ply			
		6. $ZnSO_4$	16
		Phenol	12
		Glycerine	24
		Aq. q.s.	100

of glycerine in each formula. If enough glycerine is used to dissolve all the phenol used, the mixture will be clear, whereas, the opposite is true with less glycerine. This produces a cloudy mixture. The phenol concentration remains at 24% in formulae 1 and 3, while it is reduced to 12% in all the others.

Zinc phenol mixtures are not ideal solutions for back therapy although they are extremely useful. They were the first step away from fatty-acid therapy and represented an important advance in sclerotherapy for ligaments attached to the sacrum. They are still needed for hernial sclerosis as nothing else will effectively sclerose the structures of the inguinal canal.

In the early years of my back work, an interesting case occurred in which a disabling, unstable sacroiliac sprain was not responding to routine zinc phenol therapy, using Formula 1, diluted 10 times with Xylocaine 1%. It was decided to increase the sclerosing power of the mixture by using a 2-ply concentration. Little benefit was achieved by the patient. Finally, since the ligament was not responding, 1 c.c. of Formula 1 was injected undiluted into the sacroiliac ligament. There was no immediate pain on injection and very little reaction followed. However, the following week, a dramatic and profound improvement occurred with relief of pain and improved stability.

The use of higher concentrations of zinc phenol mixtures, including stock solutions, has not been tested sufficiently because a newer concept of sclerosing solutions and the development of prolotherapy brought a halt to this testing.

Injection treatment was now divided between two camps: the adherents of sclerotherapy and the group favoring prolotherapy. Theoretically, sclerotherapy was objected to because it involved the use of injection materials that caused cellular necrosis followed by the development of scar tissue. Opposing this was the theory that the end result of scar tissue was not as desirable as the proliferation of newly formed tendon tissue.

The tendo-osseous junction was the ideal area for depositing the injected sclerosing material, and newly formed tendon tissue was thought to arise in this area. Recently there has been an extension of this theory which ascribes the origin of the newly formed tendon tissue to the periosteum of the bone at the tendo-osseous junction.

It is now theorized that relatively weaker sclerosing solutions, called proliferating agents, perform the function of stimulating tissue repair and growth, while the stronger sclerosing agents destroy tissue and get scarring as a result. The difference between these two actions is not clear because there is some cellular death and some tissue stimulation with any sclerosing or proliferative solution.

My above-mentioned early work on rabbit tendon studies reported in October 1956 (80) shows fibrous tissue proliferation within two months, following the injection of a diluted zinc phenol formula. While fibrosis was shown by histologic section, on gross examination the tendon itself was markedly enlarged and thickened. These findings were duplicated by other investigators working independently, who secured similar thickening and enlargement of the bone and tendon tissue in rabbits after injection with Sylnasol. (81) The same clinical finding resulted from two types of chemical irritants differing mainly in their sclerosing power.

With the development of prolotherapy came newer solutions, which depended for their sclerosing power on the use of fine insoluble particles in fluid suspension.

The first of these was a silicate suspension which actually contained fine particles of sand in an aqueous mixture. This material produced definite sclerosing action but had the undesirable after-effect, in some cases, of forming encapsulated tumors which were not reabsorbed. At this point, since zinc phenol mixtures produced undesirable side-effects of dizziness (due to the phenol constituent) I substituted a suspension of talc particles as an alternative injection mixture. After several years of working with these talc preparations, Gedney replaced the talc particles with pumice, and it is this mixture which is the leading agent that is used for the treatment of ligament relaxation today. His formula follows:

U.S.P. – grade, powdered pumice ½ teaspoon
4 c.c. glycerine U.S.P.
2.5 c.c. phenol

This mixture is added to 45 c.c. of 2% Xylocaine making a little more than 50 c.c. Originally this mixture was prepared without phenol, but its addition makes the solution self-sterilizing.

In using pumice mixtures, it is necessary to use a larger gauge needle in order to inject this thicker preparation. A 3½ inch spinal needle is a useful size coupled with a 5 c.c. plastic syringe.

Along with the development of suspensions of insoluble particles, the concept of prolotherapy encouraged the use of mixed sclerosing agents copied from varicose vein solutions. Thus, dextrose in 2.5 to 10% mixtures is a favorite proliferating agent. This may be used in mixtures containing propylene glycol as a vehicle. The addition of 2.5% phenol makes these mixtures self-sterilizing. Sometimes a small amount of steroid is added by some workers but this seems to retard the proliferation of fibrous tissue.

Mode of Action

The mode of action of these sclerosing materials used for sclerotherapy or prolotherapy is not completely understood. Ligaments can be repaired by the promotion of fibrous tissue, and sometimes, by bony growth. While the rabbit tendon studies indicate thickening and enlargement of the tendinous tissues, there is no study of their ultimate fate. The initial thickening in animal tissues may represent partial inflammation which may subsequently contract. There is no reason to conclude that the histologic picture in a healthy rabbit tendon will take the same course as the sprained or degenerated ligaments in the human subject.

It is difficult to conceive of a 2.5 to 5% dextrose solution acting as a specific growth factor in injured human fascia. More likely, any mild tissue irritant can provoke a series of similar inflammatory changes which could initiate repair processes. Sometimes simple needling of ligament sprains with local anesthetics acts to relax and then stimulate fascial healing.

It is in cases of severe sprains accompanied by torn ligaments, especially at their tendo-osseous insertions, that prolotherapy may sometimes be inadequate. When this occurs around the sacrum, there is often a life-long disability of a chronic nature, requiring more fibrous healing of an enduring type. Here, more potent fascial irritants like pumice or zinc solutions may be required, not only as primary injections, but repetitively on a long-term basis, perhaps for years. Where degeneration occurs, due to poor healing or other factors as yet unknown, a chronic state may take place, again requiring repeated check-ups and treatment. The whole subject of ligaments and tendon disease, the various phases in healing and non-healing of these fibrous tissues, and the kind of stimulation required to induce healing, requires much further exploration. It is important to keep one's mind open to the various modalities and not close off avenues of investigation by the use of restrictive terminology like prolotherapy. Our goal and purpose should be repair by any scientific means.

Technique

The subject of technique for injection treatment of the pelvic and spinal ligaments is a large one. Most of the injection approaches, devised by the early workers in this field, are still useful, but changes have been made and will continue to take place in a field which is still growing. The principle of the treatment is the same as in other fascial techniques. This is to inject accurately within the ligaments, a sclerosing solution at the junction of the tendon with its bony insertions.

The chief ligaments, that are most often weakened or relaxed, are the lumbosacral (supra and interspinous), iliolumbar, posterior sacroiliac (upper and lower portions), sacrospinous, and sacrotuberus. A knowledge of the technique of injection for these ligaments will handle the majority of low back syndromes due to fascial weakness.

Injections for the interspinous and supraspinous ligaments of the cervical, thoracic, and lumbar spine are vital to learn, and the technique, must be assidously performed.

Especially important is the treatment of the sacroiliac ligament as the keystone joint of the lower back. There is general agreement as to the method of injecting this important structure.

Hackett used a 22 gauge, 2½ inch needle, attached to a 5 c.c. syringe. This was inserted through the skin ½ inch from the midline, at an angle of 45 degrees, so that it entered at the angle between the sacrum and ilium. He stated that at a depth of 1½ inches the point of the needle should enter the ligament. He stressed that the needle point must impinge against bone so that some solution can be injected at the fibro-osseous junction. The direction of the needle should be changed to distribute the solution more widely. The needle should be directed more shallowly at the lower portion of the ligament, below the posterior superior spine.

In the technique of A. Gale Borden, basic landmarks for injection of the sacroiliac joint ligaments are the spinous process of the fifth lumbar vertebra and the iliac crests. The level of the L4-L5 interspace is the optimal point for entering the skin with a 3½ inch, 19 gauge needle that has a short bevel. The angle is approximately 45 degrees and the injection is started on the same side of the midline. The operator maintains gentle pressure on the skin to tense the ligamentous attachments to bone during the treatment. It is important to make contact with periosteum and bone and inject the solution as the needle is withdrawn. Approximately 6 c.c. of 8% dextrose in 1% Xylocaine, containing 0.3% phenol, will induce sclerosis of these ligaments and relief of symptoms of ligament sprain. Less than 10 c.c. will permit treatment of both sides of the joint. The point of the needle should be moved cephalad and caudad on each side of the joint.

Borden states that some patients obtain complete relief from two injections given one week apart. A series of six injections at intervals of one or two weeks is usually adequate for others. The sacroiliac joint should not be injected, only the ligament to bone attachments are treated.

In regard to the spinal techniques most workers agree that a 1½ inch needle is the proper length to use. The supraspinous and interspinous ligaments are the ones that are treated. It is convenient to treat the cervical and upper dorsal spine with the patient sitting astride a chair, and the forearms resting on the back of the chair to support the head. In this position it is possible for the operator to inject the supraspinous ligament between the spines of contiguous vertebrae.

Between the sixth cervical spine and the tenth dorsal spine, the 1½ inch needle is an advantage because the spines are longer. Above this, a 1 inch needle is safer to use in most subjects.

The solution is injected within the supraspinous and interspinous ligaments. It is safer to insert the needle up to the point of bony contact before the injection is started. More pressure will be required to spread the solution within the supraspinous ligament because it is denser. It is best to distribute the solution as the needle is withdrawn.

More than one interspinous space may be treated at one visit. It is then necessary to wait two to three weeks before retreating the same space.

The lower dorsal and upper lumbar spine is treated the same way, but the position of the patient is different. Most operators inject the lower spine with the patient lying down in the lateral position.

Three segments of spine may be treated at one time. A good plan is to alternate the injections on each side so that both sides are treated at each session. Upper and lower spinal treatments may be given at one sitting. It is also possible to treat the sacroiliac area at the same time if the patient has had previous treatment and gives a history of tolerance to multiple injections.

The other ligaments involved in low back disorders include the iliolumbar, sacrospinous, posterior sacrococcygeal, and sacrotuberous. These ligaments may also be weakened and should be injected in a similar fashion.

All of these ligaments are amenable to treatment with dextrose solutions or pumice mixtures, depending upon the experience and choice of the operator. There are other ligaments connected with the spine and pelvis that have not been mentioned. as they are infrequently affected. If the diagnosis is confirmed, and the expertise of the operator is adequate, these may also be treated.

It is unfortunate that the treatment of back disorders has been confused by the division of practitioners into two camps. This makes scientific discussion and appraisal appear contradictory, when in actuality both modalities aim at the same result. There is no real difference between the two views except in the potency of some of the solutions involved. Some solutions like pumice lie midway between the two groups, while others, depending upon the degree of dilution, can fit into either group. Thus, there is no value in creating a distinction without a difference, since fibrosis is the desired end result.

Sclerotherapy is an all embracing term which designates the art of healing diseases by the promotion of connective tissue repair, and in the process, must go through a proliferative phase. It is surprising that medical science would fragment this healing process and disturb reasoned and scientific research and documentation. It serves no purpose to encourage cloudy thinking with this unnecessary burden. The specialized name of sclerotherapy, which is universally accepted, should be retained for all phases of this therapy.

The use of sclerosing solutions for the treatment of ligament disorders has been a boon to myriads of sufferers who could not be relieved in the past. The extension and development of this mode of therapy will be a gratifying result of these injection techniques.

No one should attempt this treatment without renewed anatomical dissection and review. There is a crying need for standardized courses of instruction. This field is in an early phase with great potential for future growth.

With recognition from centers of medical education and provision for undergraduate and post-graduate training and research, this technique can become a major non-operative therapy to provide relief for this age-old universal affliction.

Chapter 24

▪ INGUINAL HERNIA, ADULT AND INFANT

With the latest improvement in hernial surgery by Shouldice (103), who reported on a new 72-hour cure, one may wonder why sclerotherapy for inguinal hernia should still be considered.

Injection treatment for hernia barely survived a critical report in September, 1937, by Burdick and Coley (104), writing in the *Annals of Surgery*. They observed, in operating on selected cases of injection failures, that it had been difficult to find the right spot to inject in order to obliterate the sac. Statistically there were 81% failures and 19% cures in their series. This disastrous, widely publicized report almost destroyed the injection method of treatment for herniae.

It was not until 1952, fifteen years later, that this unfavorable report was seriously challenged (Biegeleisen, 105). My report stated that it was unfortunate that fatty-acid solutions were popularized for this treatment. The effect of these relatively weak sclerosing solutions was to produce transitory edema of the fascia and muscles, blocking the inguinal canal temporarily.

Many physicians thought they had achieved cures after a few, or even one, injection. After subsidence of the edema, the hernia recurred because no lasting fibrosis was secured. In order to arrest false conclusions regarding hernial injections, I stressed the fact that cures depend upon permanent fascial adhesions. Fatty-acid solutions, like Sylnasol which was used by Burdick and Coley, are not sufficiently sclerosing in the inguinal canal region to produce fascial fibrosis. I recommended then, as now, a combination of zinc sulfate and phenol, with the formula described below.

This report and others like it did not undo the unfounded criticism of Burdick and Coley which was based on an erroneous concept that fatty-acid solutions, like Sylnasol, could cure inguinal herniae by injection.

It is rare in the practice of medicine that a single, unconfirmed critical report could so effectively influence medical thinking adversely that it abandoned a promising treatment method that has wide and useful applications.

In spite of the new advance in surgery by the Shouldice technique, in which patients are ambulatory the first day, and often discharged on the same day, there will always be a need for injection treatment in hernial conditions. There are groups of individuals who will always require an alternate form of treatment for the different types of hernia.

There is a group of individuals who have such a deep-seated aversion to surgery that, in spite of good health, would still reject this mode of treatment completely. Many other people would gladly accept the quick relief of modern surgery if it were not for some constitutional disorders like severe cardiovascular conditions, diabetics with advanced, difficult to control disease, and patients with diseases of the blood such as leukemia, hemophilia, and related conditions. Added to these are patients with neurologic or psychiatric problems, profoundly obese individuals, and occasionally allergic patients subject to fulminating constitutional episodes. Lastly, there are individuals who cannot tolerate general or local anesthesia.

There is another large group of hernia cases that do not respond well to surgery. These are individuals with extreme fascial weakness who show a marked tendency to recurrence either in one or more sutures or in a profound sagging of the entire operative site.

The tendency to recurrence can be early or late and may be apparent within a matter of weeks or months or be delayed for 10 to 15 years. In regard to this, we will not know if the new surgical procedure mentioned above, which gives such excellent immediate results, will bear the scrutiny of years. As yet, there is no known surgical technique which does not have some percentage of recurrence if the follow-up study is continued long enough. Statistics of recurrences following surgery are notoriously difficult to obtain as discussed previously. Many surgeons do not follow their cases for a sufficient length of time, and there is a tendency for patients who suffer a relapse to transfer to another physician, thus obviating an accurate analysis. It is easier for sclerotherapists to analyze post-injection results because they more often do periodic check-ups for this purpose.

I have had patients who were prone to hernial recurrence offer themselves for injection treatment after three or four recurrences following surgery. Some of these relapses occured in spite of transplanted fascia or other implants of various types of mesh. One patient had five operations before the surgeon himself gave up because there was no tissue left to operate on.

The demand for an alternate method of treatment for hernia in childhood and infancy will always be with us in spite of refinements of surgical technique because of the ease with which a cure can be obtained with several, or even one, injection.

There is no doubt that there still lingers in the profession's mind a stigma regarding this injection method. Closer scrutiny shows there is no scientific data to sustain this attitude. This injection method, which has a considerable background literature, has never been properly investigated, especially in its latest phases, nor have its results been properly evaluated. There is considerable ignorance regarding the subject, and even the mechanism of its operation and the histologic results are incompletely understood by many physicians.

A hernia of the abdominal cavity is a condition in which the abdominal contents emerge from an abnormal opening in the abdominal wall. The opening may be an enlargement of a normal potential aperture like a ring, or an opening may form in a weakened area where no outlet was meant to exist.

The inguinal rings are found at each end of the inguinal canal. These canals transmit the nerves and blood vessels from the inside of the abdomen to the outside where, in the male, they enter into and become part of the testicles. The canals and rings are not open normally because they are filled by spermatic cords and their accompanying structures. However, they may open if they are stretched by pressure. There are two canals in the groin, the inguinal and the femoral. The inguinal canal leads to the scrotum, while the femoral leads into the thigh from the abdomen. In the male, the inguinal canal is more often herniated while in the female, the femoral becomes the seat of hernia more often than in men. The inguinal type is far more common in both sexes and may be present at birth or appear at any age.

Both surgery and injections produce the same end results; namely, fibrous or scar tissue. In surgery, sutures hold the tissues together while fibrosis takes place. Injections produce adhesions between layers of fascial tissues, ending with a similar scar while the tissues are held together by a truss. Without the truss, injection treatment for hernia is not possible.

After a cure by the injection method, the area appears normal so that it is difficult or impossible to detect that a hernia previously existed. On the other hand, after surgery, the area is never normal again because the muscles, nerves, and blood vessels have been cut and thereby weakened. This is why in recent years permanent synthetic monofilament sutures have come to be preferred by many surgeons.

Herniae may be treated at any age by injection, but over the age of 50 the chances of a surgical success are reduced.

History

Before Bassini devised his historical hernia operation, it was customary in Europe to treat herniae by castration. This was done because no technique was available to close off the inguinal canal without injuring the spermatic cord and its adnexa. Several generations of so-called *Castrati* were produced in Italy and other countries as a result of this mutilating surgical procedure. A special type of clamp was in use for this operation.

Bassini was the first physician who conceived the idea of suturing the aponeurosis of the abdominal muscles to Poupart's ligament, thereby closing the opening in the abdominal wall while simultaneously making a new floor for the cord and its structures. This successful operation still survives today, although it has had many modifications. Injection treatment similarly closes the openings and the canal without injuring its contents.

When I began my work on herniae and published my technique in 1939 (106), there had been an immense accumulation of literature, dating back to 1835 when Velpeau used iodine to flush the hernial sac through an incision in the scrotum, which was curative. (See Table 4). As noted in this table, there had been considerable research and reporting of injection methods and solutions in the 19th and 20th centuries up to 1937, with solutions becoming more sophisticated with the passing years. When I published a detailed new technique with the use of an effective sclerosing solution that produced permanent points of adhesion, there was a considerable degree of acceptance by the profession.

The interesting background of the method is presented in Table 4, and it will be noted that much of the early work was repetitious. This historical summary shows that the technique has been in use for 100 years. It has waxed and waned in popularity during the last century.

As a result of histologic studies by Carl O. Rice (107), and improved solutions, a more favorable background has been developed. However, there is still room for improvement in technique and solutions.

A review of the older literature shows a lack of interest in detailed or standardized technique. The safety of needle angles was not sufficiently stressed in the past. The important point is the proper conception of what takes place with injection therapy. What is aimed at is adhesion between important structures as the result of fibrous tissue growth. That this fibrous growth following chemical irritation is a definite finding has been confirmed many times by surgeons operating on cases who have undergone previous injection therapy. All uniformly reported that the inguinal canal and its fascial supports were the seat of a new growth of scar tissue. Sometimes this fibrous tissue growth was so widespread and dense that it made additional surgery more difficult, but it is always possible.

TABLE 4

100-YEAR HISTORY OF INJECTION TREATMENT FOR HERNIA

DATE	*AUTHOR*	*NO. OF CASES*	*SOLUTIONS USED*	*METHOD AND RESULTS*
1835	Velpeau	3	Iodine	Flushed hernial sac through incision in scrotum; all 3 cases cured
1836	Pancoast	13 in 8 yr.	Lugol's solution. Tr. cantharides	Used syringe and cannula; all cured
1840	Jaynne		Essential oils Tr. cantharides	Special patented instrument; claimed 75% cures
1841	Heaton		Secret at first. Solution quercus albus	Special syringe and needle; disfavor of American colleges due to secrecy of method; claimed too much (100% cures [?]); only 1 injection given; patient put to bed and bandage applied
1877	Schwalbe		70% alcohol	Daily injections for about 2 weeks; patient kept in bed
1881	Warren		Quercus albus	Disciple of Heaton; only 1 massive dose given and patient confined to bed; first to describe rationale of seroplastic tissue repair; recommended painting inguinal rings and canal with solution during surgical operation (80 to 85% cures)
1892	Marcy			Discussed injection treatment in monograph on hernia
1893	Manley			Emphasized proper selection of cases
1900	Pina Mestre	15,000 (20 yr.)	Pina Mestre	Claims inguinal closed in 10-15 days (98% cures)

DATE	*AUTHOR*	*NO. OF CASES*	*SOLUTIONS USED*	*METHOD AND RESULTS*
1900 to 1932	Mayer	21,000 (30 yr.)	Zinc sulph. phenol and alcohol	First to make treatment ambulant; 98% cures; 2% cured subsequently; small doses; patient wore truss during treatment
1904	Wollerman	554	Alcohol (?)	92% cure
1907	Lannelongue		10% zinc chloride	Very enthusiastic about its use in hernia injection after noting its effect on stimulating growth of fibrous tissue in tuberculous deposits
1928	Steffen	2,775 (30 yr.)	Alcohol	One injection weekly for 1 year; no deaths in 30 years of treatment (91.2% cures)
1929	Wyss	Review of 4,632	Alcohol	3,084 follow-ups; 91% cures; no vital damage; 4% complications (abscess, orchitis, hydrocele, atrophy of testis)
1929	Hall	33	Pina Mestre	Histologic work on animals (peritoneal injections); formation of adhesions and a connective tissue barrier, thus effectively blocking and obliterating the canal; 1 failure
1930	Goldbahn		Alcohol	Reported results of unskilled injections in cases of strangulated irreducible hernias, resulting in sepsis, fecal fistulas, and deaths
1930	Jameson and Cantala	64	Pina Mestre	12 to15 daily injections; claim it is the method of choice in cases of recurrent hernia

DATE	AUTHOR	NO. OF CASES	SOLUTIONS USED	METHODS AND RESULTS
1931	Wolfe	22	Pina Mestre	Described seroplastic exudation and formation of adhesions in inguinal canal; injected into peritoneum of animals and produced plastic peritonitis; claimed cord was not injured if injected
1932	La Rochelle		Pina Mestre	Injections should supplement operative treatment, help produce internal tissue pad or truss
1933	McKinney		Phenol, alcohol, oil of thuja	Production of fibroblasts (without necrosis) in adjoining muscle tissue
1934	Larson	137	Phenol, alcohol, and thuja solution	8 injections; injection treatment suitable in 90% of cases seen (93.5% cures); no serious complication
1934	Gray	20	Mayer's solution	75% cure
1934	Bratrud	406	Tannic solution	4% recurrences with 3 final failures; animal injections; marked fibroblast proliferation, no polymorphonuclears, giant cells, or necrosis
1934	Rice	600	Phenol, alcohol, and oil of thuja, sodium psylliate	2 failures; no severe complications; histologic work on biopsy specimens from injected cases at operation shows dense adult fibrous tissue present by the forty-second day after injection
1935	Fowler	700 (5 yr.)	Tannic and gallic acids	98% cure, no serious complications; advised initial overbuilding of tissue to allow for absorption
1935	Fantus			Believes certain percentage of reducible hernia curable by injection

DATE	AUTHOR	NO. OF CASES	SOLUTIONS USED	METHODS AND RESULTS
1935	Quillin	242		210 indirect, 4 direct, 23 recurrent, 5 umbilical; work and investigation on cadaver
1935	Kretzschmar	140		Points out infections close hernial sac same as nature closes processus vaginalis
1936	McMillan	400	Thuja solution' tannic acid	8% recurrences; no serious complications
1936	Zieman and Larkowski	1	Tr. of thuja	Report necrosis of cord structures with swelling of vas after one injection
1936	Girard	174	Tannic acid, phenol, and alcohol; thuja solution; sylnasol, Pina Mestre	Series included 19 postoperative recurrences; also injected postoperative repairs with threatened weakening; claims recurrences in injected cases due to undertreatment
1936	Gordon and Gordon	5		Contradiction of injection treatment in sliding hernia; present in 1.2-1.5% of cases seen; injections, however, do not interfere with operative procedure or result
1937	Crohn		Phenol, alcohol and oil of thuja	Confirmed Rice's histologic work; no serious complications
1937	Rea			Reviewed 75 cases injected for unilateral inguinal hernia and found only 1 case of delay in libido; followed 26 cases injected for bilateral inguinal hernia for 3 years and found normal spermatic count; no sterility

It becomes important, therefore, to be able to place the needle point in the proper fascial plane by a definite, orderly, and systematic plan to secure a line of adhesions in much the same manner as after a thorough surgical operation. Some of the points of adhesion that have actually been observed at open surgery are between the aponeurosis of the external oblique and the underlying internal oblique muscle, between the conjoined tendon and the overlying fascia of the spermatic cord and external oblique muscle.

Today there is a multiplicity of surgical procedures which are still being used for curing herniae. The most recent one (108), is growing in popularity. However, the magnitude of the problem of recurring hernia has not been adequately studied, and the mechanics of the musculofascial supports have never been clearly understood. The sphincterlike mechanism of the external ring also needs further study. It has remained for the injection method of hernial treatment to stimulate interest on these important points.

In comparing both methods, one is impressed by the fact that they aim at the same end result, because they should produce adhesions in identical planes between similar structures. There are advantages to the injection method because there is no cutting or division of fascia, muscles, nerves, and blood vessels. Surgery weakens structures which are weak to begin with. As evidence of this, it is my observation that in instances where one or more recurrences take place, injection treatment has proved to be superior to surgical procedures.

Unfortunately, there is no postgraduate school that teaches this valuable therapy. The manual dexterity required with the needle and syringe is of a higher order than with the usual open surgical technique. In surgery, the operator can see and touch the tissues with which he is dealing. In the injection technique, a different kind of tactile dexterity is required because the operator must not only be aware of the structures beneath the skin and their delineation, but he has to be able to accurately find the structures or the layers between them and inject the solution in the proper plane in the correct dosage. Some accomplished surgeons were unable to acquire this kind of skill because it is a blind procedure on a different basis. The best background for acquiring this special sclerosing technique is a familiarity with the injection treatment of the other conditions described in this book. Sclerotherapy has become a field in itself, requiring the development of special skills.

Before describing the actual detailed technique, the efficacy of the injection method for direct hernia must be mentioned. This is not only in the usual direct rupture breaking through the posterior wall of the inguinal canal, but, also, for recurrent herniae which often occur through the actual suture openings. These small suture herniae are really direct ruptures, as well.

There is nothing that can deal so effectively with small direct herniae through sutures as the injection method. This is especially true for those individuals whose body structure show a high degree of fascial weakness. The only alternative to injections for these tiny recurrences is to excise the weakened part of the operative scar and do a completely new operation. This does not always succeed. Sclerotherapy has been overlooked for this valuable correction.

It should be noted that sometimes large scrotal herniae emerge from a tiny opening in the inguinal region, either of the direct or indirect type. It is comparatively easy as noted above to close this small opening effectively by judicious injection treatment concentrated in a small area.

The patients often inquire as to exercise during the treatment. With properly fitted trusses, they may exercise and continue their usual occupation. There were a number of individuals with occupations involving great muscular strain, like truck drivers, furniture movers, and others in my experience. When injection treatments were given to these hard-working individuals the results were superior to those obtained in sedentary cases. Using the abdominal muscles during the treatment aided in promoting good fascial adhesions and was encouraged.

The contraindications to injection treatment of groin herniae include irreducible or incarcerated herniae, sliding herniae, and the dangerous strangulated herniae, which are surgical emergencies.

Any inguinal hernia, to be eligible for treatment, must of course, be totally reducible. The reducibility does not always depend upon the size of the sac, as sometimes an incarcerated hernia may be small in size and yet cannot be reduced. There are individuals with large scrotal masses; that look, at first glance, as if they were hopeless, yet, with patience and the necessary relaxation, will yield to reduction. At times it has taken up to one-half hour of patient manipulation in the office before the hernial sac was finally reposited in the abdominal cavity. Occasionally it was necessary for the patient to soak in a warm bathtub for a half hour or more in order to obtain reduction at home.

Incarceration is sometimes the result of adhesions produced by incorrectly fitted trusses. It is necessary that a properly fitted truss be immediately available to hold the reduced hernia in place.

Sliding herniae are sometimes difficult to diagnose, especially by inexperienced practitioners. In those cases, it may be necessary to x-ray the bowel and clearly demonstrate that a segment of sigmoid or cecum, which anatomically does not have a full covering of parietal peritoneum, has entered the inguinal canal and descended into the scrotum. Often these non-peritonealized large bowel walls form adhesions and become totally unsuitable for injection therapy.

Sliding herniae are recognized by experienced physicians as having a different touch when the sac is palpated. The contents of the sac will feel thicker and have the characteristic feel of large bowel. This will be especially apparent upon attempt at reduction when it will be found that pushing the large intestinal walls back into the abdomen becomes a more arduous procedure. This should make the operator suspicious, and possibly indicate an x-ray for confirmation.

The alarming condition of strangulation may occur suddenly in irreducible herniae, or indeed, in any hernia which has been forced through a very small opening, usually in the inguinal canal. If the compression cuts off the vascular supply, a life-threatening situation develops rapidly. Operative intervention must be immediate because within a few hours gangrene may occur with disastrous results. Fortunately, this has never happened in my experience of many years on several thousand patients undergoing sclerotherapy for inguinal hernia.

Treatment

The fascial tissues comprising the inguinal canal will become edematous after injection by various solutions such as Sylnasol, Monolate or Sotradecol. The edema that follows their use is only transient and promotes false cures.

I have learned that the ligaments of the inguinal canal are among the toughest and the most resistant to being sclerosed successfully. In my experience the formula that follows is the only dependable sclerosing solution that will produce scar tissue here comparable with surgical repair. This formula is similar to those listed in Chapter 22 for ganglion.

Cloudy Stock Solution (Shake)

Zinc Sulphate	4 gm
Phenol	24 gm
Glycerine	16 gm
Aqua q.s. ad	100 gm

The needles used are four inch, 20 gauge, and the syringes are 5 c.c., preferably in glass. For local anesthesia 1 to 2% Procaine or Xylocaine without Adrenalin is used.

The patient is prepared by voiding to empty the bladder completely. The injection is performed with the patient lying supine on a flat table.

The location of the inguinal canal is gauged by manual examination with one finger in the external ring. On coughing, the bulge of the inguinal canal is studied. In the spare subject, the course of the femoral artery and its

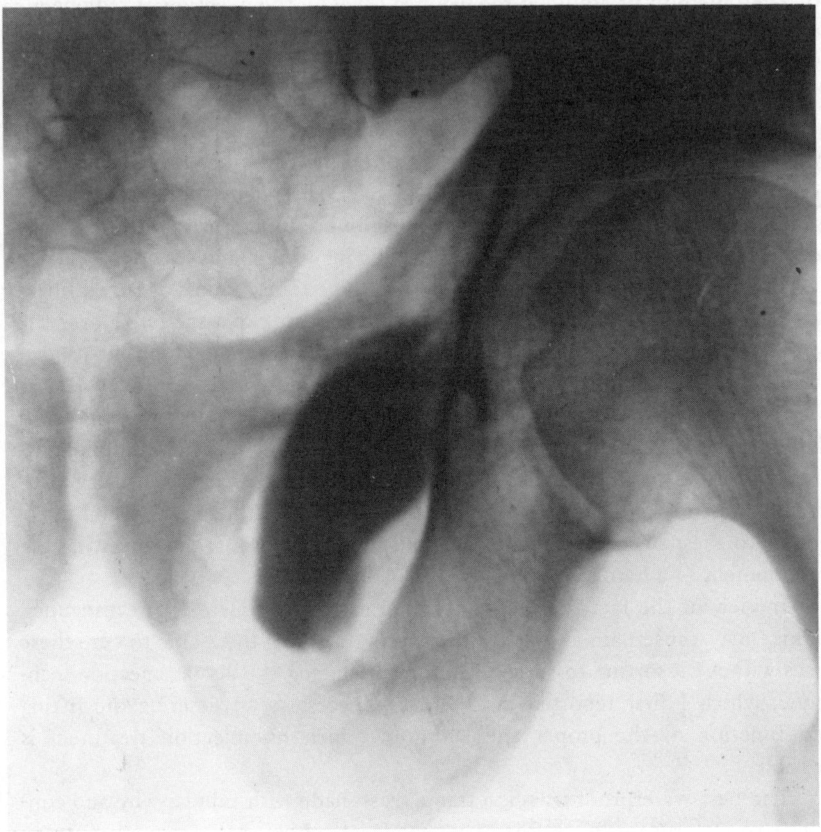

Figure 26. X-ray of bubonocele – Author's method.

branch, the deep epigastric, may sometimes be felt near the internal ring. By the aid of all these factors, the canal may be mapped out fairly accurately. An x-ray method of studying the inguinal canal by the injection of radiopaque solution will outline the canal, if it has stretched to any appreciable degree. (See Figure 26).

This x-ray method illustrates an important point in the concept of inguinal hernia. The inguinal canal is only a potential canal in the normal subject. When it begins to enlarge so that a peritoneal sac can enter it, it becomes an actual canal and is then called a bubonocele. This name, curiously enough, is derived from the condition of inguinal bubo found in connection with venereal diseases and characterized by swollen inguinal glands.

Bubonoceles are difficult to diagnose with certainty unless a trained finger can feel a tiny impulse at the external ring and an expansile bulge over the inguinal region on coughing. If in doubt, the radiopaque injection mentioned above, into the inguinal canal, will identify this potential hernia by a clear cut shadow of the canal. If no evident canal has been formed, the x-ray will simply show a fuzzy diffusing of the opaque solution without any definite outline. The value of this test lies in the fact that a canal that has just begun to stretch presents an ideal condition for the use of sclerotherapy. Several injections into the newly stretched canal should readily close it, thus arresting the development of a hernia.

In view of the fact that bubonoceles or early incomplete, indirect inguinal herniae may cause pain and discomfort, it is gratifying to be able to cure these cases without resorting to surgery. Before discussing the actual injection technique, which I first reported in 1939, it is necessary to describe the fitting and function of the proper truss without which no injection treatment is possible.

The best waterproof truss is a frame truss made with tubular wire and contains two waterproof, waterfilled pads made of rubber, while two flat buttons are attached to the rear for counter pressure. A short rubber strap holds the two buttons in place in the back. The entire truss is waterproof so the patient can bathe while wearing it. The important thing is to fit it so that the oval water pad will cover both rings, external and internal. This will keep the hernia contained within the abdomen. It is incorrect to fit the truss to press on the bulging sac only. This will make the condition worse.

Extremely accurate fitting may be achieved by experienced fitters who bend the wire frame by hand to fit closely to the contours of the patient. Similarly, while the elastic truss is usually too weak to keep a hernia reduced in the daytime, it is often ideal for sleeping when it can comfortably and effectively keep the sac reduced within the abdominal cavity.

In cases where the sac emerges close to the pubic bone, the hernia may slip out, even with a well-fitted truss unless the pad can mold itself close to and around the pubic bone. The standard water pad may not accomplish this in all cases. For this purpose a foam rubber pad covered with chamois, which has been waterproofed, will solve the problem as it is more malleable. Waterproofing may be accomplished with melted wax or suitable plastic sprays. It may also be necessary, with slim individuals, to add perineal understraps to the frame to keep the truss in place. Obese patients do not have this problem. Elastic trusses are fitted keeping the same general principles in mind.

Technique – Indirect Hernia

The internal ring is usually first injected. Classically, its location is assumed to be one-half inch above the midpoint of a line between the anterior superior spine and the pubic spine. In the presence of hernia, there may be considerable distortion. Therefore, it becomes necessary to outline the canal, as previously described. The location of the internal ring is marked on the skin with a pen.

After preliminary skin anesthesia, the needle point of the four-inch needle is inserted about 1½ inches lateral to the location of the internal ring on the prolongation of a line running through the inguinal canal. The needle is pointed in the direction of the pubic spine, and the point is depressed so that it reaches the external oblique fascia slightly above the ring margin. (See Figure 27). After penetrating the fascia, the needle is continued in the same direction through the internal oblique muscle to the traversalis fascia. The direction of the needle point here, as in subsequent injections, is always toward the pubic spine, and the angle that the needle makes with the inguinal canal is roughly 45^0. One must consider the degree of obesity present in estimating the angle of injection. The feeling experienced, in going through the skin to the transversalis fascia, is characteristic to the experienced touch. The most pronounced sensation is the "jump" of the needle point in going through the aponeurosis of the external oblique. Again, this sensation varies, depending upon the degree of firmness of the fascial structure. Experienced anesthetists compare this lack of resistance with the successful entry of the spinal canal during a lumbar tap.

Experienced operators can guide the needle through the length of the entire inguinal canal by placing the index finger of the opposing hand through the external ring into the canal. With this bimanual injection technique, the course of the needle may be folllowed through the entire canal, and the injection made retrograde on withdrawal of the needle.

The first injection is placed in the center of the internal ring. The other injections, as shown in Figure 27 are done in regular sequence. Injections two

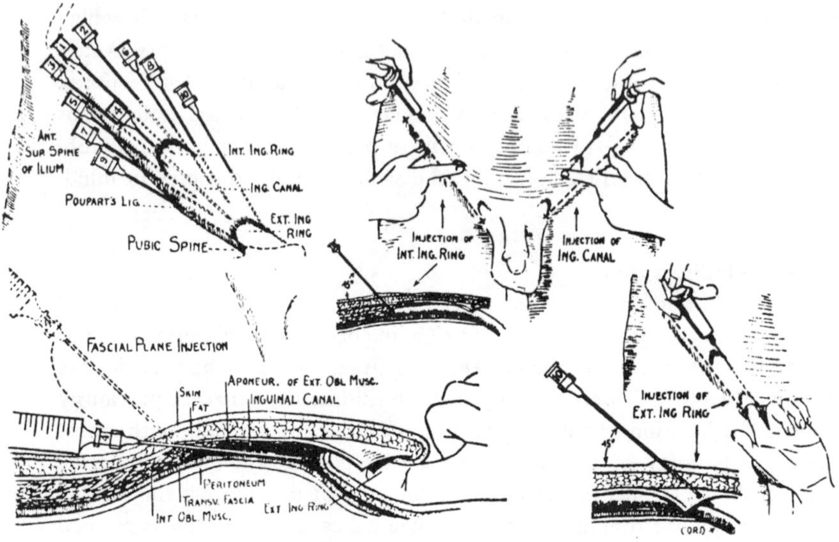

Figure 27. Injection of indirect inguinal hernia.

and three are also in the internal ring region. Four and five are placed in mid-canal, while the sixth injection goes down to the external ring in the center of the canal. Injections seven and eight are in the lower portion of the canal, while nine and ten are placed in the external ring itself.

It may be advantageous if the operator has also trained himself to treat the lower canal from below upward. In this instance, one finger is inserted into the external ring to aid in placing the needle point in the lateral margins of the ring. As a matter of fact, with a widened canal, it is possible to vary the technique so that, except for internal ring itself, all of the injections can be placed with the needle pointing upward toward the internal ring. While this technique, from below, offers some advantages to the experienced operator it is not without increased risk, as the internal ring itself cannot usually be located by the examining finger. At times, the latter technique is employed as a test to see if the canal has been successfully treated and is beginning to close.

At this point, it is necessary to discuss the placement of the operator's hands in dealing with inguinal hernia. I have found it expedient to use the following method: In treating a right inguinal hernia, I stand on the right side of the patient, invaginate the scrotum with the index finger of the right hand, and inject with the left hand.

In treating a left inguinal hernia, I stand on the left side of the patient, invaginating the scrotum with the left hand, and make the injection with the right hand. This calls for training both hands.

Some operators find it suits them better to use the same hand for injecting either side of the inguinal regions. With this method, the operator may train himself to make the injections with the left hand only and palpate the scrotum similarly only with the right hand. In doing this, he must, of course, lean over the patient to reach the opposite inguinal canal, but there is an advantage here of developing his greatest potential by concentrating these functions and training the same hand exclusively for each purpose. Whatever method is selected, it is clear that bimanual dexterity becomes an indispensable requirement of the technique.

With every injection, it is advisable to aspirate and make certain that no blood vessel has been entered. Following this, a few minims of solution are injected, and the resulting reaction is noted. After a lapse of one to two minutes, if no cramplike periotoneal symptoms are complained of, the remainder of the solution is slowly deposited. The maximum amount injected is one cubic centimeter of the zinc-phenol solution. Experienced operators generally inject the entire dose with one motion slowly, noting the patient's reaction as they proceed.

Occasionally, even in good hands, the peritoneum may be irritated, if the fluid is deposited in close proximity to it. More rarely, the peritoneal lining may actually be penetrated, and some of the solution may reach the abdominal cavity. In either case, characteristic symptoms will follow as described in Chapter 25. The operator should be prepared for this contingency which is disturbing but not harmful. The patient must be reassured that the cramps he experiences are transitory and will disappear with complete rest. Sometimes, an icebag or some ice cubes wrapped in gauze will help to allay the pain. It might also help to flood the area with 1 or 2% Procaine or Xylocaine. It is rarely necessary to administer morphine for this reaction. It simply represents temporary intestinal cramping, due to irritation of the peritoneal nerves. With experience, this will become infrequent or absent.

No case is ever complete without a few injections in the region of the conjoined tendon, as described below. This is important to avoid a direct hernia which sometimes follows and may co-exist.

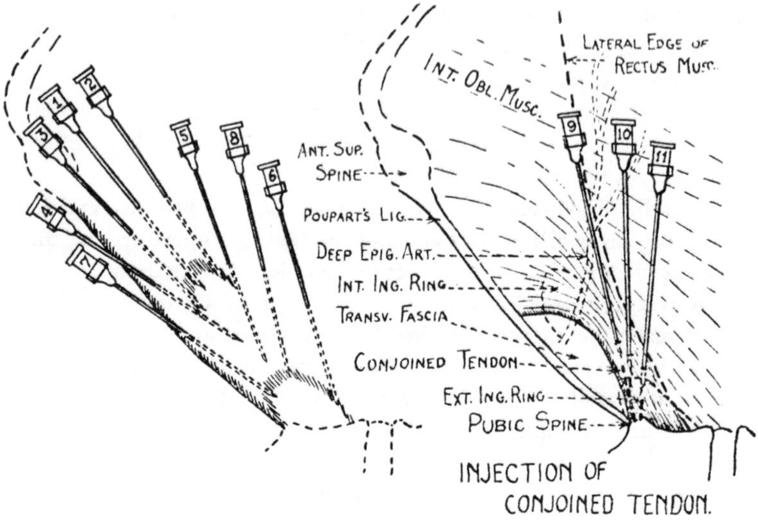

Figure 28. Injection technique for direct inguinal hernia.

Technique – Direct Hernia

There is an essential anatomical difference between the two types of inguinal hernia which necessitates a variation in technique. In indirect hernia, the posterior wall of the inguinal canal is relatively intact. In direct hernia, this wall is either weak or becomes the hernial opening (see Figure 28).

In order to secure firm and lasting adhesions, it is necessary to go outside of the canal for a safe anchoring point. What is aimed for is the formation of adhesions between the conjoined tendon, transversalis fascia, and the ligaments attached to the pubic bone in that immediate region. It is not enough to obliterate the inguinal canal in this type of hernia, as it will not cure the defect.

The technique for the upper half of the canal is exactly the same as in the indirect type. It is, therefore, advisable to do this first, to be able to concentrate on the lower region of the conjoined tendon. The reason for attacking the upper half of the canal which may be normal to begin with, is that sometimes an indirect hernia may follow the treatment. Where the type of hernia is not clear cut, as in the condition of saddle-back or combined type of hernia, the internal ring becomes more important than just mentioned.

Reference to Figure 28 will illustrate the method of attack on a direct hernia. Injections one to five are performed to close the upper half of the inguinal canal. The superior crus and the layers of the spermatic fascia are next infiltrated by the bimanual method. The cord is easily avoided. Next, the inferior crus is attacked. Using the invaginating finger as a guide, the needle point is inserted 1½ inches lateral to the pubic spine. The layers of fascia around the crus are infiltrated.

The injection of the conjoined tendon is next. In treating this important structure, the needle point is again inserted, this time 1½ inches lateral and superior to the pubic spine, keeping the syringe parallel with the lateral border of the rectus muscle. The needle is aimed at the pubic spine and actually is arrested by this bony structure after having pierced the skin, superficial fascia, external oblique aponeurosis, and conjoined tendon. When the needle touches the bone, it is withdrawn very slightly and the injection started. At this point, the needle will lie either in or below the conjoined tendon.

If the bladder is empty, as it should be, this region is a relatively safe one for injections because there are no important blood vessels or nerves in this area. The injection is made as the needle is slowly withdrawn. This is repeated several times, distributing the fluid along the area of insertion of the conjoined tendon. The operator aims to perfuse the tissues medial and posterior to the pubic spine. To make sure one is in a safe area, there should be no injection made unless bony contact has been made by the needle point at the proper level. There is surprisingly little pain during this deep injection.

Anywhere from two to six injections are made in this region, and it will be noted that induration following this treatment is often firmer than in the other portions of the canal, probably because of the sturdy attachments to the pubic bone. The last injections are made around the external ring itself. The crura are again infiltrated until it is certain that the ring is completely closed.

Technique – Femoral Hernia

This variety of hernia occurs largely in women, and while the sac emerges from the external ring region, thereby making it superficially resemble a direct hernia, careful manual examinaton will disclose that the hernia sac has entered the femoral canal and curled around upwards to emerge, as described above. In palpating to diagnose this kind of rupture, the operator must obliterate the inguinal canal above while making the patient cough. He will then note that the impulse and the sac lie in the femoral canal and generally goes upward, although it may push straight out and be felt below Poupart's ligament.

These herniae must be handled in a different fashion, as to truss and to injection technique. The pad on the truss must press below the inguinal canal and must be fitted a little lower than usual. The injections, also, are placed lower and attack not only the external ring but also the femoral canal. The conjoined tendon invariably discloses some thinning and must additionally be sclerosed. Experienced operators work around the inguinal ligament near its attachment to the pubic spine and carry the injections through this ligament, sometimes starting above and ending below, and at other times, starting below in order to end above the ligament.

It is important in this technique to know the detailed anatomy of the conjoined tendon. Its condition, especially its thickness, should be noted at the outset of every case. Sometimes it cannot be felt at all because it has been thinned out to the vanishing point. As mentioned previously, the needle point is aimed at the pubic spine and is actually stopped by this bony structure after having pierced the conjoined tendon.

Again as in direct herniae, this is a relatively safe area for injection because of the absence of important blood vessels or nerves in this space. The operator aims to infiltrate the tissues around the pubic spine. If the needle point has actually touched the bone and is then withdrawn slightly, one will be in the safe area. These deep injections cause surprisingly little pain.

A good technique for femoral hernia is aimed upwards towards Poupart's ligament and the femoral ring. The injection is started about an inch below the ligament and is carried upward in the femoral canal itself, which ends at the femoral ring. The solution is deposited as it is withdrawn for a safe injection. Naturally the femoral hernia must be completely reduced before attempting this treatment. These herniae are no more difficult to treat than direct herniae, although they are more frequently irreducible, and care must be taken before starting. If complete reduction is not possible, the case cannot be treated. Femoral hernia is primarily a female disease, as it occurs very seldom in men.

Complications.

The complication of peritoneal cramps has been mentioned previously. Two other mishaps can occur even with apparently good technique. These are sterile abscess and swelling of the cord.

A sterile abscess may occur when the reaction from the zinc phenol injection produces so much induration that it overcomes tissue resistance with partial sloughing in the area of treatment. The first sign of such a tissue breakdown is the formation of a larger than usual fusiform swelling over the inguinal canal. This does not subside within a week's time but instead remains as a cystic fluctuating and rather painless swelling. If left alone the skin may rupture and the contents are discharged through the opening. A milky white fluid is thereby evacuated and healing is uneventful. There is no acute inflammatory episode, and the whole attack is without marked inflammatory response.

In this rare development the tissues comprising the inguinal canal and its contents have undergone partial necrosis, but due to the self-sterilizing character of the sclerosing mixture, no infection has taken place. While temporarily alarming, this complication, which has happened only twice in a period of 30 years, is no barrier to continued treatment.

Swelling of the cord coverings occurs fairly often during the course of this treatment, which is to be expected, and is usually controlled by an ice pack. It is rare to inject the spermatic cord accidentally during the course of treatment, but if it happens, a different picture is presented. The patient will experience a sharp, referred pain to the region of the testicle which is a signal for the cessation of injection. It is a good idea at this juncture, using the same needle which should be left in place, to inject several c.c. of 2% Xylocaine in order to counteract the irritation of the sclerosing fluid. The operator may also flood the area with 5 c.c. of normal saline solution in an attempt to further weaken the action of the zinc phenol mixture. The reaction to the cord and its coverings to this accident will otherwise not differ from the usual one. However, if the spermatic cord has been sclerosed so that the lumen is obstructed by scar tissue, a partial atrophy of the testicle may develop.

Injury to the vas deferns, which is a slippery and movable structure, can only occur when it is fixed in place by previous treatment or disease with resultant induration or adhesions. Since the cord will not roll away due to adhesions, it may be accidentally injected during routine treatment. With experience this complication can be avoided as a transfixed cord is recognizable and special care should be used in the placing of the injections in such a case. Atrophy of the testicle has only occured two times in an experience of 30 years with this injection method.

Technique – Inguinal Hernia In Infants and Children

The problem of treatment is different for the very young because their tissues fibrose much more readily. There is also an inborn tendency for the tunica vaginalis to become obliterated after birth and when it remains patent, slight assistance often stimulates the closing. This is like the familiar example of the umbilicus, another embryonal opening which shows the same natural tendency to close spontaneously.

Everyone is familiar with the adhesive strapping treatment for this condition in infancy. This often suffices to close the opening. In severe cases the surgeon, also aware of this early tendency, simply excises the sac and ligates it while no atempt is made to suture the canal.

These facts led me in 1952 (109) to describe the injection method of hernial repair in infancy and childhood. It is an ideal method and merits more consideration, as it provides a safe and positive cure. There is no trauma to the child or his/her parents, neither is there any separation or removal from the home environment. Furthermore, there is no anesthesia problem, and the child can be returned to its normal habits almost immediately.

Treatment

This is divided into two parts, the truss and the injection. The truss is just as important as the injection. In very young infants where a truss would be impractical, strapping with elastic or plain adhesive over a gauze sponge or pad will take the place of the truss. In older children who can wear a small truss, it should be made waterproof so that they may bathe with it.

The technique of injection treatment in a general way, is the same as for adults. The needle, however, is shorter and of a smaller gauge. The usual size for the sclerosing agent is a 21 gauge 1½ inch needle. The solution used is a diluted zinc sulphate cloudy mixture described above, mixed with 1% Xylocaine. Or it may be preceded by a small injection of 1% Procaine solution.

The confidence of the child is gained by just using an anesthetic injection for the first time. This can be done with a small needle. The actual treatment is performed on the first or second visit, in the region of the internal ring. It can be located by noticing the bulge in the inguinal region produced by the baby's crying. Occasionally the structures of the cord may be palpated externally or more certainly with the invaginated finger within the ring.

A useful aid in locating the internal ring is to feel for the pulsations of the femoral artery in the child's groin. By these measures, it is almost always possible to find the internal ring. Using the 1½ inch needle at an angle of 45° with the skin, the needle point is carried to the aponeurosis of the external oblique muscle which will be encountered as a definite structure that can actually be scratched by the needle tip as an aid in its location.

Going through the aponeurosis requires an extra push and its entry imparts a characteristic jump.

The depth to which one goes is a matter of judgment. In infants, it is 1/8 to 1/4 inch depending upon the amount of muscle tissue present (in adults, ½ inch).

The proper technique is the bimanual one where the invaginating finger is kept in the inguinal canal while the other hand makes the injection. Usually the operator can insert his small finger half way into the canal. If the needle is kept pointed toward the internal ring, it will enter the canal near the structure. Now the syringe is depressed so that the needle advances inside the canal toward the external ring where it can be felt by the examining finger, near the midpoint of the canal. The injection is started as the needle is withdrawn, making it a very safe procedure. This will flood the inguinal canal with the sclerosing solution which is the same as for the adult cases. Sometimes in the very young the strength may be cut in half by diluting with equal parts of Procaine 1%. A total of .25 to .5 c.c. of solution is injected depending on the age of the child.

The reaction following injection is local swelling and redness. Some tenderness can be expected. This subsides in a day or two and most children do not complain. For greater degrees of discomfort, the application of an ice bag or cold compress will usually allay the pain. It will be noted that after the first treatment or two the hernia remains reduced although care must be exercised to keep the truss in position at all times. Bathing can be done if the truss is waterproof; otherwise the child will have to be sponged.

The number of injections will vary with the age of the child and the severity of the condition. In general, the younger the individual, the fewer injections will be needed. Up to the age of one year, one to five treatments may be given. From one to six years, five to eight treatments are advisable. From then on to puberty, the course of treatment is similar to that in adults.

The severity of the condition is not reflected by the size of the sac but by the degree of stretching of the tissues in the inguinal canal. One must also palpate the condition of the conjoined tendon and the presence or absence of the ligamentous attachments to the pubic bone. The more the ligaments have been thinned out the more treatment will be necessary.

The cardinal principle is the promotion of fascial adhesions composed of mature connective tissue, and treatment must be continued up to that point. This can be detected only one way, namely by resistance to the exploring needle. Palpation will lead to confusion as edema may feel like scar tissue. Since it may take weeks or months before scar tissue is fully formed, especially in older children, it is necessary to keep the patient under observation until this point can be proven.

It is my practice to treat young patients at intervals of one or two weeks and, after completion, to check them in one or two months. At these checkups the diagnostic injection using Procaine is made, and if no scar tissue is detected, another sclerosing treatment is given. The truss is removed only when an end result has been reached satisfactorily.

Injection treatment of hernia has never failed in infancy and childhood in my experience and, therefore, sclerosing therapy may be considered the treatment of choice in this age group.

Chapter 25

▪ RECURRENT HERNIA, UMBILICAL HERNIA

Most hernial recurrences are direct in type; the failure of an entire operative site is comparatively rare. Fortunately, in many instances the operative wound gives way at only one or two sutures. This creates several small direct herniae which are uniquely simple to close with sclerotherapy. A second surgical operation, however, requires excision of at least part of the first scar and another dissection and repair. If this was the only benefit offered by this injection technique for hernia, the method would still deserve a permanent place in medicine. This important fact is not emphasized enough and is relatively unknown to many.

Surgeons themselves could very well use this simple method of repair for many of their hernial failures. Even in those cases where repeated operations have failed on the same individual, the final result is still a series of small direct herniae. The repair, is often unbelievably simple, and will now be described.

Technique

The solution employed is the zinc phenol formula listed in Chapter 24. A proper truss must be worn. This is described in the previous chapter for inguinal hernia. In the female, the same solutions and truss are required.

The operator must first identify the hernial openings. These are usually small, globular protrusions from sutures that have failed to unite the tissues. The examining finger will readily reduce the small sac which is made up of peritoneum with other fascial membranes.

After reducing the sac, the operator can now locate and anesthesize the margins of the opening. This is done with 2% Xylocaine and a 23 or 21 gauge 1½ inch needle. It will be noted that the margins of the small ring are formed by comparatively thin tissue which is easy to penetrate if one is not careful. This is of the utmost importance when making the actual sclerosing injections.

Since we are not dealing with the actual inguinal canal, a long needle is unnecessary. The rule to follow is that the length and gauge of the needle should be the smallest consistent with the thickness of the opening. In most cases, the opening is just below the skin layers.

The zinc phenol solution is carefully injected into the margins of the entire ring. It will be found that a few minims will suffice for each point chosen. It is often possible from one insertion of the needle to inject almost half of the margin around the opening. One should be on the lookout for peritoneal reactions.

When treating these direct herniae, the operator is dangerously close to the peritoneal cavity. This is not found in any other type of hernia. If the needle passes the margin of the ring, even slightly, some of the solution will enter the abdominal cavity to cause intense cramping. Sometimes the tip of the needle does not penetrate the margin of the ring but only gets close to the peritoneal layer. The injected solution will then distend the tissues causing pressure on the lining. This may cause a less intense peritoneal response.

The typical peritoneal reaction can never be mistaken for anything else once it is witnessed. The patient develops an intense abdominal cramp which sometimes doubles him up and makes breathing difficult. Some patients describe the pain as agonizing, and certainly all of them become extremely apprehensive. However, the operator must, by his behavior and demeanor, convey a strong reassurance to the patient that the pain is only momentary and will spontaneously subside within a few minutes. It may be allayed somewhat by the immediate injection of Xylocaine, 2%, into the affected margin of the ring. Occasionally morphine or Demerol will be useful to provide quick and complete relief. Once allayed, the pain does not recur.

With experience, it will be possible to make the injection safely by carefully stopping short of penetrating the margin. The necessary dexterity and appropriate gauging of the depth of the tissue will be learned rather quickly. The number of injections that will be required to close the opening depends upon its size, number of openings, the character of the scar tissue, and the patient's response to treatment.

With a single small opening, one treatment may be all that is needed to sclerose the ostium. If the operator feels that it is desirable to further strengthen the tissue that fills in, he can do this readily by injecting into the area that is healing to cause a stronger sclerotic reaction and scar. The same principle holds true if there are several little pouches to close. I have found only rare instances where this effective treatment does not work properly. Sometimes the injections have to be repeated before closure is final. It seems to be ideal for this condition.

As noted above, there is a group of individuals with exaggerated fascial weakness who do not respond to any kind of hernial surgery. These are people who have undergone three or more operative repairs including special grafting techniques. Some of them have had wire mesh or fascial grafts, wire clips or metal sutures which hold where they are placed, but develop recurrences adjacent to the areas that are repaired. Some of these cases were beyond ordinary help because surgeons would no longer operate on them. Injection treatment in these patients was the only treatment possible because of surgical rejection.

There is another group of post-operative recurrences which involve part of the area or sometimes the entire area (dehiscence). If part of the operative site fails to unite, it may be in the form of a larger direct hernia or, anatomically, it may be a partial relapse of the previous inguinal hernia. Some of these relapses are mixed types and cannot be classified in the usual sense. The partial failure of the operation may be due to various factors such as poor technique or infection. The operator must utilize the methods described in the previous chapter in addition to the technique just outlined for small direct pouches. These infrequent types of major surgical failure may do better with injection treatment than by excising the entire operative site and doing a completely new operation. The injection method does not cut any nerves or actual ligamentous structures but merely causes fibrosis and scar tissue. Since these relapsing areas often occur in previously weak tissue, it is important to avoid further weakening of the fascia by additional surgery.

Lastly, there is a group of individuals with marked fascial weakness who do not respond well to either surgery or sclerotherapy. Injection treatment may transform these patients from a difficult hernial problem to a simplified case. By repeated injections at suitable intervals, it will become possible for the sufferer to improve sufficiently so that a light elastic type of truss may make him comfortable although he has not obtained an actual cure.

Umbilical Hernia

This will be discussed under two headings, the infantile type and the adult.

Infantile Type

All obstetricians and most family physicians are aware of the fact that umbilical hernia in infants can be cured simply by strapping the umbilical area with adhesive tape. First the hernia is reduced by pressure over the umbilicus. Maintaining this pressure, the operator fastens strips of adhesive over the depressed umbilicus in order to pull both sides of the hernia together. Three or four strips of tape may be needed to completely efface the protrusion. Instead of adhesive strips, elastic adhesive may be used and replaced every few days until the two edges of the hernia adhere firmly to each other.

Since the umbilicus normally has an inherent power to grow shut by natural coaption, it becomes an easy matter for the physician to assist this pronounced normal tendency by strapping the two sides together. This treatment rarely fails, but in the event that closure does not take place, it becomes an easy matter to carefully inject a drop or two of sclerosing fluid, diluted five or ten times, in the margins of the hernia. This will effect a cure if the umbilicus is then pulled together with adhesive.

Adult Type

Umbilical herniae may develop in the adult as the result of increased intra-abdominal pressure. These ruptures are most often partially incarcerated so that only a bubble of sac containing some omentum is present. This is usually quite readily reducible. In an occasional case, the hernia may grow to considerable porportions but this is unusual. All cases require a special abdominal belt-like truss for treatment. This should consist of a hard rubber flat button attached to an elastic band going around the waist. They are then amenable to sclerotherapy.

Since they are direct, herniae injection should be performed around the fascial openings with great care to avoid spilling any fluid into the peritoneal cavity. This accident will also cause the severe abdominal cramping typical of peritoneal irritation as described above.

The technique is to use a 1 inch needle or possibly 1½ inch size for the preliminary local anesthesia of 2% Xylocaine which should be followed by the standard zinc-phenol mixture as in inguinal herniae. The margins of the ring forming the opening in the umbilicus or the fascial openings are injected so that the entire circumference is treated either immediately or in sections. The hernia must be reduced completely and kept in this condition throughout the injection period of treatment.

Afterwards, the reduction must be maintained by the properly fitted button truss mentioned above. The plastic button should be flat for if pointed it will widen the opening at the umbilicus. Sometimes these buttons are rounded in the center which is also objectionable as it may prevent the opening from closing.

Treatments are given at weekly intervals until enough scar tissue has formed for permanent closure. These herniae are relatively easy to close as the openings are often small. Occasionally, a large rupture with a wide annulus may be difficult to bridge and require considerable tissue proliferation for effective healing.

It is a matter of judgment for the operator to decide whether the treatment in these cases is worth attempting.

Surgery can always be done in the event of failure by injection. The flat button truss must be worn for several months after successful closure. It is usually not required for sleeping during the later half of the treatment. Even if the hernia is reduced in size, or just appears in the upright position, it may be worthwhile to render this nonoperative treatment for comfort if not complete cure.

Chapter 26

ANGIOMA, HYPERTROPHIED TURBINATES AND EPISTAXIS

The extension of sclerotherapy for angiomas was one of the earliest I attempted. The first cases were in infants and children exhibiting angiomas of the lips, face, and body.

It was not generally known then that many so-called "strawberry lesions," if left alone in infancy, would spontaneously regress within a few years without any treatment at all. Even today, when the cherry-red growths are located on the lips, it is difficult to persuade anxious parents to wait a few years and see what happens. Since sclerotherapy is relatively simple, I have occasionally favored early treatment. This helps to avoid the lip distortion that sometimes follows later treatment, because more mature scar tissue may develop. However, with protruding vascular growths on the body rather than on the face or lips, waiting for natural regression is better practice.

Employing cryotherapy in the form of carbon dioxide snow for these lesions may produce evident scarring, as will occur after dessication. Sclerotherapy, therefore, is the preferred method and should always be considered.

Angiomas may be venous, arterial, or capillary in type. The cavernous angiomas, which are usually venous, are the ones more commonly found in infancy and childhood. The treatment to be described will produce obliteration with minimal or no scarring. The solution of choice is quinine and urethane diluted with 2% Procaine or Xylocaine in the proportions of 2 to 1, 1 to 1, or 1 to 2. The 1 to 1 (50%) solution is the one most commonly used. It is advisable to begin with the weakest solution and advance to the stronger mixtures as needed. Large lesions often require stronger mixtures and repeated injections to effect a cure.

Treatment is ordinarily subcutaneous and not intravenous. However, if a blood vessel is entered, one minim of solution may be attempted and the effect studied as in varicose veins. The technique must be modified depending upon the location of the birthmark.

If the lesion is on the body, from 1 to 5 minims are injected subcutaneously into the tumor mass until visible blanching occurs. It is advisable to select a point outside the lesion and, using this as a center, make radiating injections into the entire area. One should attempt to avoid necrosis and subsequent scarring by judicious estimation of the amount injected.

The rule of injecting until there is some blanching is the guide to correct treatment. If the elevated strawberry mark is large or deep, it may be necessary to carry out the treatment in two or more sessions.

Sometimes slight scarring will be seen in the early healing stage, but this often gradually becomes less noticeable in infants or even disappears completely with time and growth.

Lesions on the lip or other parts of the face are treated more carefully and with the weakest solutions that will produce the desired effect. Thus, the 1 to 2 mixture mentioned above might be the preliminary or test injection. The result of this will again be a good guide to the subsequent treatment. It is sometimes necessary to end up with the stronger 2 to 1 mixture of quinine and Xylocaine.

The needles for this facial treatment should be a smaller gauge, beginning with 27 gauge and following with the finer 30 gauge. A 25 gauge for larger or denser growths may be required.

Flat Angiomas

Flat angiomas which have a variety of names including Nevus Vasculosus or "port-wine" stains, while not common, are so disfiguring that they can never be forgotten once seen. Previously, when present on the face, the afflicted individual had to go through life with a terrible handicap.

It is only recently, in 1968, that Solomon, Goldman, et al (110) published their results of the laser treatment of port-wine hemangiomas. This hitherto incurable, disfiguring, livid stain on the skin was now, for the first time, amenable to treatment. While the results were about 60% good or excellent, scarring did occur, in some instances, around the lips in a small percentage of cases. Not all of the lesions were removed completely, because only lightening of the discoloration was achieved in the less successful results. Nevertheless, where it was effective, actual cures were obtained for the first time in a disease that had resisted the many and varied attacks upon it by physicians in the past, including tatooing therapy.

Laser therapy, while not achieved by the injection of sclerosing solutions, is related to sclerotherapy by virtue of the action of the argon laser rays, which are selectively absorbed by the red cell hemoglobin and converted into thermal energy with resulting superficial vascular thrombosis and coagulative necrosis. The overall picture resembles granulation tissue and varies from case to case. Therefore, the inclusion of this treatment in a manual of sclerotherapy is not unjustified.

I have had a dramatic and successful result in a woman with an enormous port-wine stain, treated by sclerosing injections of 1% Sotradecol. The lesion covered the lateral surface of the entire lower extremity from the buttock down to the ankle, and disappeared completely after two years of treatment. This case is described in more detail in Chapter 27 which deals with future applications of sclerotherapy. It cannot be recommended for routine treatment until further studies are made.

Hypertrophied Turbinates

This condition in allergic states or hypertrophic rhinitis can be treated so simply that, while it is in the province of otolaryngology, it yields so well to sclerotherapy that it can be described here.

The older and more usual treatment for reduction of enlarged turbinates in office practice was by means of chromic acid beads or electro-coagulation. While these established methods are highly successful in reducing the size of the hypertrophied tissue, they sometimes have the annoying after-effect of drying the mucosa of the nose. Injection with a sclerosing solution, on the other hand, produces satisfactory shrinkage without noticeably affecting the mucosa of the turbinate mass. The results are very rapid and the relief obtained often dramatic.

The solution of choice is quinine lactate in a saturated solution which is about 16% concentration. The area is first anesthetized by swabbing with Procaine-Adrenalin mixture. Using a 30 gauge needle, 0.25 c.c. of quinine lactate solution is injected into each of four points along the inferior turbinate. Intravascular injections should be avoided. A few minims of sodium morrhuate solution have been used for the same purpose.

The nares are plugged with cotton for a half hour after which the cotton may be removed. In about three weeks, if sufficient shrinkage has not been obtained, the treatment may be repeated.

Epistaxis

Common nasal bleeding frequently is spontaneous, especially in older individuals suffering from hypertension. Often it follows trauma or is seen as a post-operative complication.

The classic site is Little's area and, if this is the source, the control is very simple. Sometimes, however, the source is in some other part of the nose and control of massive bleeding may become a life-saving procedure. Every doctor is familiar with the occasional case of epistaxis which does not respond to the usual, often frantic, methods of hemorrhage control.

The most dangerous situation exists when the bleeding is in the back of the nose and is due to the rupture of a small arteriole. Here the ingenuity of the physician is taxed to the utmost and, sometimes, the only control is surgical ligature of one of the arteries feeding this area.

In most cases, however, whether the bleeding is from the classic site or further back, if it is recurring despite the usual methods of relief, they become suitable cases for sclerotherapy.

Some familiarity with nasal work is necessary to locate the hemorrhage and secure proper exposure for the injection. The patient should be in a sitting position with the head tilted slightly forward to keep the blood out of the larynx. First, epinephrine (1:1000) solution, or other astringent in cases of hypertension, should be applied to the bleeding area by cotton tampon or gauze pack. It is also advisable to apply a 2% solution of Xylocaine on a cotton pledget to the septal area involved. This is left in place for 10 minutes. At this time, one can note the blood vessels more clearly against the blanched mucosa. A point is selected, as low down as possible, a fraction of an inch in front of the bleeding point. Here a cotton-tipped applicator containing alcohol is gently rubbed and the needle inserted, submucosally. An injection is made to blanch the affected venules until 0.25 to 0.5 c.c. of sodium morrhuate has been injected. A tuft of cotton is left in the nares to exert slight pressure. It will be found that in most cases the injection of the sclerosing solution produces an immediate edema which seals the venules effectively and stops the bleeding. Subsequent tissue reaction to the chemical irritation adds to the initial effect until permanent fibrosis takes place. The proper choice of needles and syringes must be made so the operator can reach the entire length of the septum. Difficult, deeper injections should be made only by those familiar with nose and throat techniques.

If the area can be visualized and injected in this fashion, most nasal hemorrhages can be promptly arrested. The general practitioner dealing with the usual hemorrhage near the anterior nares can perform this simple procedure himself.

Chapter 27

■ FUTURE APPLICATIONS OF SCLEROTHERAPY

The future of sclerotherapy is almost boundless because the results obtained are as good as, and sometimes better than those following surgery. The extensions of sclerotherapy described here are an example of this trend and are exciting to contemplate.

Some of the techniques described here have been attempted experimentally but are not in actual practice because the methods need more study. The rest of the chapter consists of hypothetical new techniques which, while not attempted before, have a firm basis for their proposal. Together they embody an extension of research that should be most productive and important for the future.

The healing process in the human body has been studied extensively but there are still elements of disagreement as to the role of the cells involved. In spite of an information explosion regarding an enormous diversity of studies, often unrelated to any central theme, basic cellular changes are still not completely understood. From the simplest degeneration like cloudy swelling, to other more complicated cellular pathologic changes, the nature of the degenerative changes remains unclear. Other examples of this lack of knowledge are found in our studies regarding the growth and development of the human embryo. We do not know what the limiting factors are that control the growth process, both orderly and disorganized.

In discussing the action of sclerotherapy which stimulates the repair process, we are aware again of basic inadequate knowledge. The body heals largely by fibrous tissue. In routine surgery, diseased tissues are excised or divided and then the raw surfaces are sutured together by various techniques for union. This is often by scar tissue, and the suturing or stapling is merely a mechanism to hold the tissues together until the scar secures them properly. The sutures and staples are then often unnecessary and are either removed or left in place permanently.

Similarly, in sclerotherapy, tissues are deliberately irritated, injured, or destroyed chemically and are subsequently replaced by fibrous tissue. By either method, surgical or injection, the end result is a scar, but a study of the two processes points up some interesting differences.

When cells are cut, their cellular contents are strewn into the tissues where they send out chemical signals that stimulate wound repair. The exact nature of the cellular components that are released is not completely understood. If we could identify the biological stimulants it would be possible to isolate and use them so that we could program body healing and direct its course. We have not yet reached this stage and, therefore, we must rely upon the primitive technique of injuring tissue in order to promote healing. This is already under attack by some workers who object to tissue destruction, preferring tissue stimulation instead and who call their process prolotherapy in contrast to sclerotherapy. This has been discussed previously.

More work is needed to understand the mechanism of fibrous tissue repair following chemical irritation. In the case of sclerotherapy does the chemical death of a cell release the same hormones and cellular fluids as following the mechanical destruction of a cell by the surgical scalpel? We don't know. What we do know is the clinical fact that the strands of fibrous tissue formed after surgical excision or incision are denser and longer lasting than the scar that follows chemical injury of identical tissue. It is as if the tissue itself gets a signal that makes it aware of the need for stronger reconstruction following an incision made by a scalpel. Whether there is a neural element, as well, because the knife cut may have severed nerve fibers along with blood vessels, or whether a special signal is sent out because of the immediate prolapse or sag that follows incision, is pure conjecture at this point. It is fortunate that the division of ligamentous or muscle tissue is followed by an especially dense scar, because this counterbalances the deleterious effect of cutting across important supportive tissues. On the other hand, a chemical injection, while producing a less dense scar, is often preferred because blood vessels and nerves have not been cut. One must see the whole picture in proper perspective to evaluate the differences between the two kinds of therapy.

The ideal method of repairing the human body would be to isolate and inject the actual hormones that promote the formation of a satisfactory scar without cutting or further traumatizing the tissues involved. This would greatly reduce the amount of surgery performed to correct the body's ills.

The response of organ structures and mucosal tissues is on a different order. Here, we are dealing with endodermal tissues, and the repair that takes place following treatment, while it is fibrotic, is different. The fibrosis that takes place after varicose vein injections has been previously described and is characteristic for blood vessels, but differs from organ structures.

The proposals that I am submitting below are not a complete list but merely indicate some of the exciting possibilities that lie ahead with sclerotherapy. This list is not in any order because there has been no systematic exploration of the extension of injection methods for human disease. First I will describe methods already attempted and then hypothetical suggested techniques which have a logical basis for their exploration.

Methods Attempted Requiring Further Study

Prostatic Hypertrophy

The injection of substances into the prostate gland was first introduced in the United States in 1917 by Townsend, Valentine, and Cano. It was previously practiced in foreign countries. Grant (111) reported 500 cases in 1934 in which the prostate gland had been injected with 1% Mercurochrome. Grant recommended this treatment for those cases of chronic prostatitis which failed to improve after months of treatment by massage, heat, and other conservative treatment. The type of prostate found most suitable for this treatment was the enlarged, boggy type, which showed secretions after massage.

In order to obtain satisfactory results, it was necessary to inject the seminal vesicles. These are usually infected, in this type of prostatic enlargement, and were injected with the same 1% Mercurochrome. This was done by performing a vasotomy and injecting in a retrograde fashion.

Some of the other drugs that have been used are Metaphen (1:2500 solution), a weak solution of organic iodine, Sylnasol 5%, and other mild sclerosing agents. These injections produced scar tissue in the gland.

Penn Riddle (112) believes that prostatic enlargement is due to varicose veins, causing venous stasis of the prostate. This in turn produces benign hypertrophy of the prostate gland. Varicose veins of the urinary bladder are often noted in association with hypertrophy of the prostate. Riddle asserts that the production of venous and lymph stasis is an expected consequence by the altered physiology in the region due to the varicosities. These veins may be present in the bladder, prostate, and rectum, and contribute to the venous stasis and hypertrophy.

The hypertrophied prostate causes poor emptying of the bladder and more impairment of the venous circulation. In order to correct a vicious cycle, the prostate must be decompressed. This may be accomplished by standard surgical methods or by sclerosing treatment. Sclerosing therapy is followed by fibrous tissue, which upon contraction expels stagnant pools of lymph and serum.

Technique of Injection

In Grant's method, both vasa deferentia are injected. The bladder is filled with sterile water with the patient lying on his back, and after local anesthesia, a one-inch incision is made into the upper portion of the scrotum on each side. The exposed vasa are injected using a fine 26 gauge needle, inserted into each vas, and 5 c.c. of 1% Mercurochrome is injected into each side. The skin is sewed up, and the patient is put into the lithotomy position for the next injection.

The prostate is palpated through the rectum, and an 8 inch, 20 gauge needle is introduced through the skin above the border of the rectum and passed downward until it can be felt by the finger in the rectum. The needle can then be guided to the left lobe of the prostate without puncturing the rectum.

After passing through the prostate capsule, it should be pushed further, about 3/8 of an inch, into the body of the gland. At this point 5 to 10 c.c. of Mercurochrome is injected.

The needle is now withdrawn to a point outside the capsule of the prostate and reinserted into the right lobe where the injection is repeated. It will take considerable pressure to push the plunger of the syringe and force the fluid into the gland. The gland can be felt to distend as it is injected. After the injection, the prostate is massaged by the finger in the rectum, and the bladder is then emptied by the patient.

The prostate may also be injected by the rectal or urethral route, but the perineal route above is the best technique.

Riddle's method is to give small injections of sclerosing solutions every week for four weeks. He makes this an ambulant office treatment. To expose the vas, he uses local anesthesia of the scrotal skin and the vas area. He employs four injections, and if necessary, two additional treatments for the lateral lobes.

The above workers claim that the prostate gland is reduced in size by this form of sclerotherapy. Lovelace and Emmett (113) have confirmed the shrinking by injecting dogs' prostates with Sylnasol.

Grant claimed excellent results in 500 cases as did Townsend, who also reported the same number of cases. Three other investigators, O'Connor, Ladd, and Greenslade (114) also reported on this treatment, warning of possible bladder neck obstruction in gonorrheal prostates. However, this is infrequent and does not contraindicate treatment in these cases.

In spite of the background of sclerotherapy for this important condition, this method has not been investigated in recent years, probably because of the difficult techniques involved. With the newer and safer solutions available today, further investigation of this promising treatment is called for as it can simplify the management of hypertrophy of the prostate.

The widespread existence of prostatic hypertrophy in an aging population has been increasing and is bound to grow still further as advances in geriatrics are made. If successfully developed, a good technique will render inestimable benefits to a large body of sufferers who now must submit to sensitive and precarious surgery. It should be possible with improved technique to eliminate the dangers of hemorrhage and impotency that often follow surgical correction. In time, this technique will probably become well established.

II. Port-Wine Stains

This disfiguring skin blemish, while not common, is so striking that once seen it can never be forgotten. Years ago, following the successful application of sclerotherapy in cavernous angiomas, I was led to consider using this method on flat angiomas. My research was a preliminary study involving 15 individuals who exhibited this lesion on the face. While my results were encouraging, I will not describe them at this point because the research was halted when the more successful laser therapy was developed (115).

Laser therapy for port-wine stain of the face is now an establsihed form of therapy for this disfiguring disease. While it cannot be used in all cases because of its complications, these can be eliminated by spot testing prior to actual treatment. Cosman and other early workers have secured 59% of good or excellent results in selected cases.

It did not seem worthwhile for me to continue injecting flat angiomas on faces when the new laser modality achieved such early, good results. However, upon reflection, I feel that the injection of sclerosing solutions in port-wine stains of the face should be continued because a large segment of cases are not appropriate for this treatment with laser rays.

I can now describe my experiences with the treatment of flat angioma on the lower extremities. At first I attempted to treat these skin lesions by undercutting the skin with long tenotomy knives, which were introduced under the skin that had been anesthetized. These knives were swept in an arc subcutaneously to cut through and free the whole skin layer from the underlying tissues. It is significant of the tenacious chronicity of these stubborn blemishes that this radical attack did not modify the lesion. It was then decided to treat a series of patients with widespread port-wine stains by the injection of sclerosing solution. This was done in the following fashion.

The area to be treated was subdivided by a skin marker into patches measuring 2 x 4 inches, rather than attempting the entire blemish at one sitting. Using a 4 inch, 20 gauge needle, the previously outlined area was injected with 1 or 2% Procaine or Xylocaine in a special technique.

With the flat bevel of the needle kept upright, the anesthetic was gradually injected, as the needle was advanced to its maximum length. It was relatively simple to stay in a subcutaneous plane as the injections continued. Furthermore, it was possible to cover the entire area with Procaine or Xylocaine from one puncture point. By fanning out from this point, the 2 x 4 inch quadrangle could be completely covered by the solution. This was a painless procedure because the anesthetic was injected as the needle was advanced. With each fanning thrust, the needle was withdrawn back to the original puncture point before it was thrust forward at a new angle. When the entire area was anesthetized, the needle was withdrawn completely.

Following this, a syringe containing 5 c.c. of the sclerosing solution and carrying another similar 4 inch needle was again introduced through the same skin point, and another series of radial fanning injections were made. This time, however, the solution was injected while withdrawing the needle, making for even distribution of the 1% Sotradecol solution. The importance of getting a uniform spread of the sclerosing solution is obvious because pooling or concentrating the medication at one point might produce skin necrosis. I never observed any sloughing with this technique and believe that a stronger concentration or indeed other sclerosing solutions are possible medications.

After treatment, the area became red, mildly inflamed, and sometimes a little swollen. This was easily controlled by five minutes of cooling with ice. This stopped uncomfortable symptoms.

I began my study by treating port-wine stains of the thigh and leg. Early responses to this treatment were rather inconclusive because what was obtained was an uneven, blotchy lightening of the wide-spread lesions. I continued some of these cases for months, in several cases up to one year. The treatments were given every few weeks. As the treatments dragged out, both the patient and I became discouraged and the treatment was halted.

In one outstanding case, where the hemangioma easily covered one-third of the skin area of the lower extremity, treatment was continued for practically one year, and the patient vanished with only the mottling result described above. This individual returned after three years for check-up treatment of her varicose veins and to my surprise the port-wine stain had completely disappeared. I cannot state whether the entire year's treatment was necessary, but further study of this method is obviously indicated.

III. Wrinkles and Sagging Tissues

I have treated many women with sagging dependant folds of skin or wrinkling in the upper portion of the inner thigh regions by sclerotherapy.

This is not an uncommon finding in women over the age of 40 who have lost weight or otherwise have less subcutaneous fat from other causes. The women have brought these folds to my attention during varicose vein therapy, feeling, perhaps, that they are somehow related to the varicose vein condition.

Over the years, I have attempted to shrink the skin and the underlying subcutaneous areas by the injection of sclerosing solutions, notably 1% Sotradecol. The results have been encouraging in some cases and indifferent in others. The problem has been that progress by this therapy is slow and difficult to prove. I have often felt that with persistence many of the milder cases of adipose wrinkling would have responded to this therapy. This technique is as follows.

Anesthesia is secured with 1% Xylocaine, which is injected subcutaneously as in the case of flat angioma, but a little deeper. The needle is a 4 inch, 20 gauge size, and the bevel is kept up during the injection.

An area is selected measuring about 2 x 4 inches, and the anesthetic is introduced as the needle advances to its preferred length but is not withdrawn. Instead, the syringe is removed at this juncture and another syringe containing 1% Sotradecol is attached, and an injection is made as the needle is withdrawn, care being taken for an even distribution of the sclerosing solution to avoid pooling of too much medication at any point. This is important to prevent sloughing.

It will be noted that the area treated will become red and inflamed soon after the treatment. The patient may complain of burning and heat. Ice packs should be applied immediately for relief as the irritation will quickly subside with the cold pack.

This treatment may be repeated every week and several areas may be treated at one time. The skin and subcutaneous treatment will show, after several treatments, increased thickening and resistance to the injection indicating beginning fibrosis which will ultimately shrink.

Mild cases of wrinkling will improve with this therapy. Sagging folds require much more sclerosing. Skin tissues are notoriously slow in response to sclerotherapy, and caution must be observed not to render these treatments too closely together. After a few injections, an area under treatment must be given one to two months rest to permit the development of fibrosis. Patience is needed for success.

IV. Corns, Warts, and Papillomas

An oily solution of Vitamin A has been found efficacious for removal of corns (clavus) of the foot. Many podiatrists and physicians have been employing this method since 1950. There is a possibility for the development of a standard sclerosing technique for this disease of the skin. Such a solution should produce more uniform and consistent results than the oily vitamin preparation.

Warts present a fascinating topic for discussion. In skin clinics around the country many dermatologists advise what seems to be an old wives' nostrum; namely, the use of saliva directly applied to the wart by the patient as a treatment. Physicians have almost facetiously advised their patients to "spit" on the wart every day, and they would disappear after two weeks of this therapy. To everyone's amazement, this has occurred often. The explanation is not simple. One can theorize that the digestive enzymes found in saliva may actually be digesting either the cornified epithelium or the viruses which are supposedly causing the wart.

Aside from the above therapy, which can hardly be termed scientific, warts and papillomas of the skin may be routinely injected with a sclerosing solution like sodium morrhuate for satisfactory therapy. The injection must be made in the base of the growth where it arises from the skin. Usually 1 to 3 minims will suffice for a small growth. If there is a pedicle involved, injection must be made into the attachment of the pedicle to the skin.

V. Injection Treatment of Urethral Stricture

Injection treatment for urethral stricture now has a background of successful therapy for the past 25 years. Working independently, this method of injection was developed by urologists in a manner similar to the technique I described for lymphedema of the leg mentioned earlier in this book.

Since the thickened area of a urethral stricture may be considered a form of local induration, similar to that found in lymphedema of leg tissues, the two methods have a basic relationship with each other. Furthermore, they both respond to infiltration with isotonic solutions, enhancing this relationship. An impressive series of patients who responded favorably to injection technique has been collected. Early workers used a solution containing cortisone which was injected through the cystoscope, after locating the stricture by x-ray of the urethra and bladder. Each patient received a short series of these treatments but had to be cystoscoped for each session.

The wall of induration is self-defeating in the body's healing mechanism. It is known as the wall of Boom when it is found around the margins of old ulcers of the leg. (116) In this wall, after injections, new capillaries and lymphatic channels develop which aid in the healing process. This indurated wall is found around the edges of most inflammatory lesions of the body. It is nature's attempt to limit infection and inflammation, but often it mitigates against circulation and healing. I have found that piercing it with injections of normal saline relieves the induration and often prevents it from contracting by scar tissue which could have a harmful effect.

Investigators were aware of this mechanism when they began using this injection technique for what had previously been considered an intractible, permanent, dangerous scar around the urethral canal of the male and occasionally the female.

There is room for an alternative technique whereby the injection is made externally through the perineum. This would eliminate the traumatizing cystoscopic approach. Normal saline could be substituted for cortisone. This area is a fertile field for investigation of a condition which has often been life threatening. It deserves more study and much wider usage. I have seen results which are dramatically successful when all other measures fail.

Hypothetical Methods Not Yet Attempted

The following theoretical applications, while not attempted as yet, have a credible foundation for their proposal. They illustrate the vast potential for this mode of therapy, and, undoubtedly, these and many other conditions will ultimately yield to the syringe and sclerosing solution.

I. Rectal Polyps and Cancer

In my work on the injection treatment of internal hemorrhoids, I have often injected rectal polyps either inadvertently or deliberately along with the piles themselves. These polyps, at the time, seemed grossly unaffected by malignant changes. I have no doubt that many other physicians treating hemorrhoids have found it difficult or impossible to treat this condition without including rectal polyps.

While none of the polyps showed any indication of neoplastic changes, it is possible that beginning new growth had already started in some of these polyps. It is interesting to note that no anal or rectal cancer followed injection treatment in my large series of hemorrhoid cases for the past 30 years. Is it justifiable to speculate that some of these polypoid masses had beginning new growth which was effectively sclerosed by the injection treatment? Certainly none of these cases were stimulated by the treatment to develop cancer in these areas.

From this conjecture it is fair to assume that there is a potential for curing cancer in early cases beginning in rectal polyps. In validating this theory, one should control any investigation by making careful biopsies of the polypoid tissues before and after treatment. Since the rectal area is a frequent locus for cancer, it becomes a most important research venture because of the ease and amenability of treatment.

II. Spot Reduction

A promising field for development is the use of sclerosing solutions for localized areas requiring cosmetic improvement. Mention has been made of a technique I have used for the elimination of wrinkles and skin folds at the upper, inner thigh of menopausal women. Extending this therapy to the face and body is a natural afterthought. Thus, sagging, wrinkling and puffiness on the face or neck could, theoretically, be relieved by constrictive or tightening sclerotherapy.

In much the same manner as the plastic surgeon tightens the skin of the face, present solutions or future improved reagents could be utilized for this purpose. It is difficult to conceive of large areas on the abdomen or pelvic girdle succumbing to extensive sclerotherapy. However, this desirable result may be within our grasp if fibrosis can be promoted in the future by the use of hormonal development of sclerosing solutions.

III. Ptoses – External and Internal

Among the conditions affecting the human race adversely are sagging defects like pendulous breasts, dropped kidneys, cystocele, rectocele, and the various ptoses of the uterus. These are now corrected surgically by appropriate techniques. Great skill is required in breast repair and some of the other procedures, but it would be useful if an injection technique could be developed which would strengthen the fascia that supports these organs.

In early or minor instances of these conditions, it is theoretically possible to develop a sclerosing technique to ameliorate these prolapses, thereby avoiding surgery with all its problems. Thus, Cooper's suspensory ligament of the breast could be dealt with to prevent further sagging. With improved technique it may one day be possible to shorten this ligament and correct the condition.

IV. Thyroid Enlargement

The exciting possibility of injecting enlarged thyroids has been appreciably diminished since the advent of anti-thyroid drugs. However, there is still a narrow area in thyroid therapy which might be more effectively and minutely controlled by sclerotherapy. The treatment of hyperthyroidism has been highly developed into an intricate multiple mechanism, with only a little room left for sclerotherapy. Nevertheless, conditions like colloid goiter or other enlargements still require surgery and remain a field of exploration for sclerotherapy. Drug sensitivities, allergies, and uncomfortable side effects also leave room for an alternate method of treatment. Finally, for individuals who are not suited for surgery, an alternate method would be welcomed.

V. Glaucoma

Glaucoma has been treated by surgical excision of a wedge in the iris diaphragm of the eye. This opens up an avenue of lymphatic flow which has been blocked by the disease process. Medically, glaucoma is treated by the instillation of pupillary constricting solutions like Pilocarpine (0.5 to 4%) in the eye. This assists the flow of lymph in the eye.

There is a constant lymphatic diffusion within the eyeball due to the ingress and egress of lymph fluid through vascular channels in the eyeball. In the condition of glaucoma, there is a block of varying degree which cuts down the outflow of lymph from the eyeball. This takes place in the cribriform plate, which behaves like a filtering mechanism for the lymph fluid that is bathing the eyeball. The lymphatic flow is in constant operation in the healthy eye. It does not take much obstruction or interference to cause increased pressure leading to blindness.

Because lymphatic obstruction in the leg can be relieved by subcutaneous infiltrating injections which open up new pathways for lymphatic flow, it occurred to me that a parallel method might assist the lymph flow within the eyeball. There is a possibility that the obstruction in the cribriform plate, which is also of a lymphatic nature, could similarly be assisted by a very delicate microscopic injection technique using normal saline. Within the eyeball where pressures are of paramount importance, it is obvious that solutions cannot be injected without making some compensation for the withdrawal of a similar amount. This would be necessary for homeostasis in the eyeball. However, even simple needling without injection might provide some measure of relief. Work in this area of even a simple nature could well be productive of enormous gains, as glaucoma is a major threat to eyesight in many individuals.

VI. Basal Cell Epithelioma

This menacing skin condition, while not completely accepted as a true skin cancer by some physicians, is nevertheless, capable of occasional metastasis.

Dermatologists have developed a highly effective method of diagnosis and treatment. This consists of skin biopsy followed by curettage or excision of the skin lesions if they have basal cell pathology.

While the majority of basal cell epitheliomas on the face can be successfully treated in this fashion, there are instances where lesions close to the eye, lips, or other precarious locations, are not amenable to surgical removal without causing disfigurement. It is for these cases that investigation of treatment by sclerosing injections may be rewarding. In view of the successful injection treatment of other skin blemishes, notably raised angiomas, I feel that basal cell lesions comprise another logical area for investigation.

Depending upon the size and developmental stage of the skin lesion, a few minims up to 0.5 c.c. of 3% Sotradecol may be tested by injecting the base of each individual epithelioma. In the usual fashion, biopsy should preceed the experimental injection to determine the size and depth of the basal cell growth. The object should be to destroy or sclerose the skin growth. Other solutions may also be tried.*

In the region of the eye, needles should be appropriately small, 27-30 gauge. Research on the treatment of basal cell lesions, if successful, may lead to the application of sclerotherapy for other new growths. Thus, even if the new growth is within the body and can only be reached by open operation, sclerotherapy may be useful for early cancer in locations that are not easily amenable to surgery. The exploration of sclerotherapy for the treatment of cancer has not really begun, but it should be started because of its great potential for the future.

VII. Artificial Skin for Leg Ulcer

This material which is undergoing intensive investigation and development was first introduced in the United States for the treatment of injuries resulting from exposure to fire. Most of them required urgent treatment because fire had destroyed a large portion of their skin.

Homografts enjoy considerable use in the treatment of massive burns. Whether the source is a live donor or skin is obtained from a cadaver and used immediately or after preservation in a skin bank, homografts are in short supply. In the absence of immunosuppressive agents, homographs are commonly rejected.

---

*I have recently successfully treated a basal cell epithelioma of the wrist (to be published).

Heterografts, particularly porcine skin grafts, are commercially available for burn treatment and have also been used successfully for leg ulcers.

Reconstituted collagen membranes have also been employed by several investigators. Collagen has been extracted from animals, purified, and converted to films which have been used as wound dressings as early as 1943. A large body of synthetic membranes has been investigated in the treatment of burns. This research has not so far led to the solution of the problem of a skin substitute. The work is going on with collagen components at the present time. The latest finding is that the pore structure of swollen collagen membranes can be preserved by a freeze-drying process which has a greater potential for skin replacement. This is the material which should be experimented with for the grafting of large skin ulcers in the lower extremities (117).

Conclusion

In conclusion, some of the hypothetical instances where the expansion of sclerosing procedures may take place in the future have been described. This necessary expansion will take place more readily if teaching institutions and hospitals will be more aware of the potential of this new field of medicine. Especially important is a teaching program to educate physicians in the art of employing the procedures described in this book.

The growth of sclerotherapy will further reduce the morbidity and mortality of many diseases.

▪ BIBLIOGRAPHY

1. Sherman RS. Varicose veins anatomic findings and an operative procedure based upon them. Ann Surg 120:772-784, 1944.

2. Biegeleisen HI. Unilateral enlargement of the lower extremity accompanying varicose veins with Roentgen studies of "deep venous block". Amer J Roent Vol XLII, Nov 5, 1939.

3. McPheeters HO. *Injection Treatment of Varicose Veins.* FA Davis Co 1938.

4. Biegeleisen HI. Telangiectasia associated with varicose veins, treatment by a micro-injection technique. J A M A 102:2092-2094, 1934.

5. Biegeleisen HI. Unilateral enlargement of the lower extremity accompanying varicose veins with Roentgen studies of "deep venous block". Amer J Roent Vol XLII, Nov 5, 1939.

6. Biegeleisen HI. *Primer of Sclerotherapy; Injection Treatment.* Froben Press 1944.

7. Higgins TT, Kittel PB. Injection treatment with sodium morrhuate. Lancet i:68-69, 1930.

8. Biegeleisen, HI. Evaluation of sodium morrhuate therapy in varicose veins. Surg Gyn & Obs 57:696-700, 1933.

9. Biegeleisen HI. Fatty acid solutions for the injection treatment of varicose veins: evaluation of four new solutions. Ann Surg 105:610-615, 1937.

10. Biegeleisen HI. Two fatty acid solutions for the injection treatment of hernia. Am J Surg 37:413-417, 1937.

11. McPheeters HO, Lufkin N. Histologic studies on injected varicose veins. Surg Gyn & Obs liv:511-517, 1932.

12. Gautier A, Mourgues L. Compt rend Acad d Sc Par cvii:110-112, 1888.

13. Ghosh S. Indian J M Research viii:211-215, 1920.

14. Cutting RA. J Lab & Clin Med xi:842-845, 1926.

15. Biegeleisen HI. Evaluation of sodium morrhuate therapy in varicose veins. Surg Gyn & Obs 57:696-700, Nov 1933.

16. Fegan WG. Continuous compression technique of injecting varicose veins. Lancet 2:109-112, 1963.

17. Biegeleisen HI. End results of surgery for varicose veins: twenty-eight-year study of 200 cases. NY St J M 60, 15:2386-2393, 1960.

18. Sherman RS. Varicose veins anatomic findings and an operative procedure based on them. Ann Surg 120:772-784, 1944.

19. Fegan WG. Continuous compression technique of injecting varicose veins. Lancet 2:109-112, 1963.

20. Biegeleisen HI. The diagnosis of phlebitis in varicose veins with the aid of the sedimentation rate. Ann Surg 99:661-667, 1934.

21. McPheeters HO. Anderson JK. Injection treatment of varicose veins and hemorrhoids. Fa Davis Co., Phila. 1943.

22. Hume M. Blood coagulation in deep and superficial thrombophlebitis. Arch Surg 92:934-936, 1966.

23. Szczepanski M. Investigations on the blood coagulation and the euglobulin clot lysis time in superficial thrombophlebitis. Hemostase VI:247-254, 1966.

24. de Takats G. Amer J Surg xviii:26, 1932.

25. Biegeleisen HI. The diagnosis of phlebitis in varicose viens with the aid of the sedimentation rate. Ann Surg 99:661-667, 1934.

26. Biegeleisen HI. Rapid injection treatment of varicose veins. Clin Med 8:10, 1961.

27. McPheeters HO. Injection treatment of varicose veins. FA Davis Co 1938.

28. Sullivan JM. Varicose veins in pregnancy. Wise MJ 49:291, 1950;

29. Biegeleisen HI. Phlebitis in varicose veins. Lancet 904, Apr 1936.

30. Biegeleisen HI. Varicose veins, a chronic disease; evaluation of twenty years experience in treatment. NY St JM 53:963, 1953.

31. Biegeleisen, HI. Phlebitis in varicose veins. 904, Apr 1936.

32. Shank PJ. Ohio St JM 44:477, 1948.

33. Peyton EW, Loop FA. Saphenous phlebectomy for varicose veins during pregnancy. Amer J Obs & Gyn 58:318, 1949.

34. Sullivan JM, Walske BR. Thrombophlebitis: an evaluation of various methods of treatment. Amer J Surg 79:355, 1950.

35. Hamilton HG, Pittam RF, Higgins RS. Active Therapy of Varicose Veins in Pregnancy. South MJ 42:608, 1949.

36. Titus P. *Management of Obstetrical Difficulties.* CV Mosby & Co. Phila 130, 1940.

37. Adair FL, Stieglitz EJ. *Obstetric Medicine* Lea & Febiger Phila 1934.

38. Solomons E. Treatment of varicose veins in pregnancy. Irish JM Sci 296:353, 1950.

39. Samuels SS. *The Diagnosis and Treatment of Diseases of the Peripheral Arteries.* Oxford Univ Press NY:260, 1936.

40. Sherman RS. Varicose veins anatomic findings and an operative procedure based upon them. Ann Surg 120:772-784, 1944.

41. Fegan WG. Continuous compression technique of injecting varicose veins. Lancet 2:109-112, 1963.

42. Lofgren KA. Long-term results after vein surgery. Mayo Clin Proc 49:115, 1974.

43. Varicose veins. Editorial, Lancet 2:391, 1959.

44. Biegeleisen, HI. End results of surgery for varicose veins: twenty eight year study of 200 cases. NY St J M 60:15:2386-2393, 1960.

45. Tunick US, Kling DH. New method of treating chronic ulcer of the leg. Am J Surg 13:524, 1931.

46. Cruikshank W. The anatomy of the absorbing vessels of the human body. G. Nicol London ed 2:148, 1790.

47. Halsted WS. The swelling of the arm after operations for cancer of the breast: elephantiasis chirurgica, cause and prevention, Bull. Johns Hopkins Hosp 32:309, 1921. Replantation of entire limbs without suture of vessels. Proc Nat Acad Sc 8:181, 1922.

48. Reichert FL. The recognition of elephantiasis and of elephantoid conditions by soft tissue roentgenograms, with a report on the problem of experimental lymphedema. Arch Surg 20:543, 1930.

49. Homans J, Zollinger R. Experimental thrombophlebitis and lymphatic obstruction of the lower limb. Arch Surg 18:992, 1929.

50. Drinker CK, Field MD, Homans J. Experimental production of lymphedema and elephantiasis as a result of lymphatic obstruction. Am J Physiol 108:509, 1934.

51. Castellani A. Elephantiasis nostras (non-filarial elephantiasis). Proc Roy Soc Med 27:519, 1934.

52. Kinmonth JB, Taylor GW, Harper RK. Lymphangiography: a technique for its clinical use in the lower limb. Brit M J 1:940-942, 1955.

53. Kinmonth JB, Bryant JS, Gruber D, Townes PL. Primary lymphoedema. Clinical and lymphangiographic studies of a series of 107 patients in which the lower limbs were affected. Brit J Surg 45:1, 1957.

54. Kinmonth, JB. Lymphangiography in man. A method of outlining lymphatic trunks at operation. Clin Sci 11:13-20, 1952.

55. Yune HY, Harris PF, Vix VA, Klatte EC. Direct injection mediastinal lymphography, animal experiments. Radiology 92:817-823, 1969.

56. Brincker H, Ingstrup H, Jensen TS, Skjoldborg H. Lymphographic demonstration of cisterna chyli trauma: Intralymphatic injection of patent blue violet during operation. Acta Radiologica:Diagnosis 8:461-464, 1969.

57. Kinmonth JB, Bryant JS, Gruber D, Townes PL. Primary lymphoedema. Clinical and lymphangiographic studies of a series of 107 patients in which the lower limbs were affected. Brit J Surg 45:1, 1957.

58. Drinker CK, Field MD, Homans J. Experimental production of lymphedema and elephantiasis as a result of lymphatic obstruction. Am J Physiol 108:509, 1934.

59. Torgerson WR. Auchincloss operation: preliminary report. Porto Rico J Pub Health & Trop Med 6:411, 1931.

60. Biegeleisen HI. Lymphedema occurring with varicose veins, treatment by injection. Arch Derm & Syph 33:689-696, 1936.

61. Tunick US, Kling DH. New method of treating chronic ulcer of the leg. Am J Surg 13:524, 1931.

62. Oliver RF, Grant RA, Kent CM. The fate of cutaneously and subcutaneously implanted trypsin purified dermal collagen in the pig. Brit J Exp Path 53:540-546, 1972.

63. Yannas IV, Burke JF. Design of artificial skin: basic design principles. J Biomed Materials Res 14:65-81, 1980.

64. Biegeleisen HI. Unilateral enlargement of the lower extremity accompanying varicose veins with Roentgen studies of "deep venous block". Amer J Roent Vol XLII, Nov 5, 1939.

65. Mahorner HR. Ochsner A. New test for evaluating circulation in venous system of lower extremity affected by varicosities. Arch Surg 33:479-492, 1936.

66. Biegeleisen HI. Telangiectasia associated with varicose veins. JAMA 102:2092-2094, 1934.

67. Madden JF. Generalized angiomatosis (telangiectasia). JAMA 102: 442, 1934.

68. Biegeleisen, HI. Telangiectasia associated with varicose veins. JAMA 102:2092-2094, 1934.

69. Biegeleisen HI. Telangiectasia associated with varicose veins. JAMA 102:2092-2094, 1934.

70. Biegeleisen HI. Biegeleisen KP. Fascial weakness: a new clinical syndrome. Clin Med 78: 14-17, 1971.

71. Chvapil M. *Physiology of Connective Tissue.* Czech Med Press, Prague 123, 1967.

72. Chvapil M. *Physiology of Connective Tissue.* Czech Med Press, Prague 123:1967.

73. Ayer JP. Connective Tissue Res 2:33, 1964.

74. Svejcar J, et al. Clin Sci 24:325, 1963.

75. Hisaw FL, Zarrow MS. Vitamins Hormones 8:151, 1950.

76. Chamberlain WE. Proc Dalif Acad Med pp 41-96, 1937-38.

77. Hisaw FL, Zarrow MS. Vitamins Hormones 8:151, 1950.

78. Hisaw FL, Zarrow MS. Vitamins Hormones 8:151, 1950.

79. Wilson R. Amer J Med 23:434, 1957.

80. Biegeleisen HI. New injection treatment of low back syndrome due to weakened ligaments with new solution. NY Phys & Amer Med 47:3, 1956.

81. Borden AG. Some investigational aspects of prolotherapy in animals and man. Clin Symp Prolotherapy Assoc San Francisco 1969.

82. Biegeleisen, HI. Biegeleisen KP. Fascial weakness: a new clinical syndrome. Clin Med 78:14-17, 1971.

83. Hanes GS. Treatment of rectal prolapse by hypodermic injections of hydrochloric acid. Trans Amer Proctol Soc pp 112, 1928.

84. Gabriel WB. The principles and practice of rectal surgery. HK Lewis, London p 62, 1932.

85. Potter EB, Wellman JM. Alcohol injection for prolapse of rectum. JAMA 100:1891, 1933.

86. Hanes GS. Treatment of rectal prolapse by hypodermic injections of hydrochloric acid. Trans Amer Proctol Soc pp 112, 1928.

87. Graham AB. The use of injections in the treatment of fissure in ano. Trans Amer Proctol Soc pp 43, 1926.

88. Gabriel WB. *The Principles and Practice of Rectal Surgery.* Lewis HK, p 72, London 1932.

89. Cutler EC, Zollinger R. The use of sclerosing solution in the treatment of cysts and fistulae. Am J Surg 19:411, 1933.

90. Biegeleisen HI. Sclerotherapy for pilonidal cyst. Am J Surg 44:622-625, 1939.

91. Dzondi CH. On congenital fistula of the trachea. Schwetsche & Son 1829, Brit Rec Obs Med & Surg 1, 1848.

92. Biegeleisen HI. Sclerotherapy for pilonidal cyst. Am J Surg 44:622-625, 1939.

93. Biegeleisen HI. Biegeleisen KP. Fascial weakness: a new clinical syndrome. Clin Med 78:14-17, 1971.

94. Mixter WJ, Barr JS. Ruptured intervertebral disc with involvement of spinal canal NE J M 211:210-215, 1934.

95. Ghormley RK. An etiologic study of backache and sciatic pain. Proc Staff Meet, Mayo Clinic 26:457-463, 1951.

96. Gardner E. Blood and nerve supply of joints. Stanford M Bull 11:203 1953.

97. Scuderi C. Diagnosis and treatment of backache from the standpoint of the general practitioner. J Okla St M A pp 191-197, 1954.

98. Biegeleisen HI. Sclerotherapy (sclerosing injection treatment). NY Phys & Amer Med 45, 3:28, 1955.

99. Gedney EH. Disk syndrome. Osteo Prof 18:12, 11-15m 38-46, 1951.

100. Hackett GS. Joint ligament relaxation treated by fibro-osseous proliferation. Charles C. Thomas, Illinois, 1956.

101. Manucher JJ. Treatment of herniated lumbar disk syndrome with chymopapain. JAMA 243, 20:2043-2048, 1980.

102. Gedney EH. Hypermobile joint. Osteo Prof 4:9:30-31, 1937.

103. Shouldice EE. Surgical treatment of hernia. Ont Med Rev 4:43 1945.

104. Burdick EG, Coley BL. Injection method of treating hernia. Ann Surg 106:322, 1937.

105. Biegeleisen HI. The treatment of inguinal hernia in infancy and childhood by the injection method; 13 years experience. NY Phys & Amer Med 38:Nos 5-6, 1952.

106. Biegeleisen HI, Tartakow IJ. Technique of the injection treatment for inguinal hernia. Surg 5:202-216, 1939.

107. Rice CO. Hernia, its cure by the injection of irritating solutions. J Iowa St M S 1936.

108. Shouldice EE. Surgical treatment of hernia. Ont Med Rev 4:43, 1945.

109. Biegeleisen HI. The treatment of inguinal hernia in infancy and childhood by the injection method: 15 years experience. NY Phys & Amer Med 38:5, 6, 1952.

110. Solomon H, Goldman L, Henderson B, Runfield D, Frazer M. Histopathology of the laser treatment of port-wine lesions. J Invest Dermatol 50:141, 1968.

111. Grant O. Treatment of chronic prostatitis by injection. J Urology 33:640, 1935.

112. Riddle P. Injection treatment. Saunders WB 1940.

113. Riddle P. Injection treatment. Saunders WB 1940.

114. Riddle P. Injection treatment. Saunders WB 1940.

115. Cosman B. Clinical experience in the laser therapy of port wine stains. Lasers in Surg & Med 1:133, 1980.

116. Tunick US, Kling DH. New method of treating chronic ulcer of the leg. Am J Surg 13:524, 1931.

117. Yannas IV, Burke JF. Design of artificial skin: basic design principles. J Biomed Materials Res 14:65-81, 1980.

▪ INDEX

Printed in Canada